Urologist's Guide to

PENIS ENLARGEMENT

MICHAEL KAPLAN MD

Disclaimer

This book is solely for informational and educational purposes, and is not intended for medical advice. Before starting any exercise program you should always check with your personal physician. The use of any herbal supplement, exercise, device, injection or surgery for penis enlargement is controversial, and does not have widespread approval of the medical community. There are potential risks with any form of intervention, and readers are advised to use caution. Just as one would ease into any exercise program, one should approach penis enlargement in the same manner. This book is not intended to diagnose or treat any medical condition. Rather than to dismiss all forms of penis enlargement, the author has attempted to present the potential benefits as well as side affects of the available options, and allow the reader to make their own judgment.

This book contains information from multiple sources, the publisher makes no warranties, either express or implied, as to the accuracy or fitness for a particular purpose of the information or advice contained herein. The publisher wishes to make it clear that this book is for information purposes only, as a supplement to one own judgment. This book is not intended to diagnose, treat, cure or prevent any disease. Neither the publisher nor author shall be responsible or liable for any loss, injury or damage caused to any person or property arising in any way from the use of this book. The information presented in this book is not intended as a substitute for the advice of a medical professional. If you have any concerns about your health, we strongly advise you to discuss it with your personal healthcare practitioner as soon as possible. Statements in this book have not been evaluated by the Food and Drug Administration.

INTRODUCTION

Working as a private practice urologist for over twenty five years I had the opportunity to examine many thousands of men and their genitalia. I can't tell you how many of these examinations started with men "shaking out the rust" so as to awaken the sleeping giant. They were subconsciously transiently increasing the size of their penis for inspection. Why did these guys care what I thought about the size of their penis? This was occasionally followed by a comment such as "I know its small, but it gets the job done". Sometimes I would hear "Is there anything you can do to make it bigger? " Most urologists don't believe in male enhancement, although it is commonly accepted that weight loss, particularly with attention to loss of central obesity can result in the appearance of larger external genitalia. (About one half of the penis is actually internal.) In response to these frequent concerns, I would usually make a reassuring comment such as "you have nothing to worry about, you're fine." I would also fall back on a reference to the fabled bell shaped curve, and explain that most men fall within that curve, and as long as that is the case, size has little to do with satisfying one's partner. For many years I told my patients this with absolute confidence, knowing that size did not matter, unless one desired a career in the porn industry. This supreme confidence based upon medical science was shattered one day when I saw an episode of Sex in the City in which Samantha presented her unique female view. She summarily rejected the advances of an otherwise well qualified suitor based upon his inadequate penis size. Her loyal fiends all agreed with her decision. They agreed that size does indeed matter!

Around the same time, a host of male enhancement products were popularized, and surgery for penile enlargement became widely available. In fact, at one time, a product known as Enzyte was one of the most popular over the counter medications in America. Advertisements for penis enlargement became commonplace in sports pages throughout the country. In spite of the apparent desire for many men to enlarge their penises, the science lagged behind the market. Most of the over the counter medications were based on little if any science. Similarly, there were many documented surgical misadventures resulting in mangled penises, disappointment, lawsuits, and occasional deaths.

This book is written in hopes of helping men find answers to a subject with very little legitimate literature. There are countless urological texts, journals and conferences on every aspect of urological disease, but almost no attention paid to two of the most common questions asked of urologists every day. Is my penis big enough? What can I do to make it bigger?

TABLE OF CONTENTS

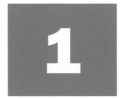

Size

Worries About Penis Size

Although many men spend a great deal of time observing and worrying about their penis, there is often great reluctance to ask their friends or their doctor the types of questions that are really on their minds. One of the great questions that is often left unasked is the question of size. "How do I match up to other guys?" Almost every man has compared his penis to other men in the locker room. About half of all men have genuine concerns about the size of their penis.

Men tend to be much more concerned about penis size than women, although there clearly is a subset of women who find size to be extremely important. If you are in this group of approximately 50% of all guys that have some concerns about the size of their penis, it's reassuring to know that you're not alone. It's also reassuring to know that men tend to put much greater emphasis on this then do most women.

Why do men worry about size? Is it because of their concern about being able to satisfy their sexual partner? The reality is that the most important ingredient for achieving a satisfying sex life is the ability to satisfy one's partner. In other words, if your partner is having a great time, odds are, so are you. That does not necessarily have a strong correlation to size in most relationships. The reality is that most women are not concerned with the size at all. However, as we will learn, for some women (about 20%), this is of critical importance. Suffice it to say, the size of a man's penis is not the cornerstone of a healthy relationship. Many men equate their ability to bring a woman to a screaming, heart-pounding orgasm as being directly correlated with the size of their penis. They equate their sexual prowess and desirability as measurable quantities determined by size. On the other hand, most of their target audience, women, have a very different perspective.

SECTION 2

To What Are You Comparing Your Penis?

The first penis (other than their own) that most guys remember seeing is their father's. This is most unfortunate, as Dad's penis is relatively monstrous in size compared to a young boy's. This image may haunt the young man for years, remembering in an exaggerated form, the size of this relatively huge organ. This comparison can be the start of years of anxiety over the ability to attract and keep a mate.

The Porn Affect

With the explosion of the internet and the ready availability of pornography, men are found comparing their own penises to those of porn stars. The porn industry does not feature men with normal-sized penises. In fact, the average porn star is packing 8 inches plus (the Industry standard). If the only other men you ever saw play basketball were Lebron James and Steph Curry, you'd probably get discouraged and give up the game.

Most heterosexual men never see another man with an erection other than in some form of pornography, and, hence, the disconnect between reality and perception. There is a very specific subset of pornography which does feature men with very small penises or micropenis. In these films, women mock and humiliate the unfortunate individuals. This only serves to reinforce the myth that only large organs can satisfy women, and increase a fragile guy's insecurity. They also lead guys into thinking that most other guys are hung much better than they are.

SECTION 3

Predicting The Size Of A Man's Penis

The absolute most important influence regarding the size of a man's penis is genetics. This genetic influence does not seem to correlate very well with any other genetic factors with the exception of a mild correlation with height. There is no strong evidence suggesting a significant difference in penis size based on race. The science goes very much against some popularly held beliefs. Similarly, there is no correlation between the size of a man's penis and his shoe size or the size of his hands or fingers. There is evidence that the lower the ratio of the index finger to the ring finger, the longer the penis.

One obvious factor that can influence the perceived size of a penis is bodyweight. Certainly, the addition of central obesity can result in the appearance of a smaller penis. As a man gains weight, the penis can be surrounded and enveloped by fat and look much smaller. It has been stated that the loss of 35 pounds of weight in an obese patient can result in an apparent gain of 1 inch in the penis.

Low-dose systemic testosterone has been used to treat micropenis in boys prior to puberty, but is not effective in adults. After puberty, administration of testosterone does not affect penile size. As such, oral medication alone does not change the size of the penis. There is little scientific evidence that the many pills or supplements that claim to change the size of a penis have much efficacy, as a stand alone treatment. However, they may be helpful when used in conjunction with exercises designed to stretch the penis.

There are conflicting reports regarding the change in the size of man's penis with age. Some reports do indicate that the penis becomes smaller with age. In addition, the corpora cavernosa likely become less compliant with age and likely expands less with age. That means that men's penises expand less with erections as they get older.

Even though there are very few reliable tools that correlate with penis size, that does not mean there is nothing available to help the handicapping process, as evidenced by the Predicktor, an Android App that utilizes measures that some believe have been shown to predict penis length. This includes such things as height, sexual orientation, and finger- length. This was developed by a family physician in Toronto, Dr. Chris Culligan.

SECTION 4

Does Size Matter?

A man's perspective:

Most men wish that they were bigger. We are naturally competitive. Men want to be stronger, smarter, richer and better looking then other men. That is the way we are wired. Size is not the most important factor for most men, but to give penis size no importance is not realistic.

The size of a man's penis may influence their own body image or sense of sexual confidence but does not influence their own personal ability to enjoy sex. While 75% of women do not reach orgasm through penile-vaginal intercourse, over 98% of men have an orgasm every time. The remaining 2% of men have a poorly understood condition called anorgasmia.

If a man's primary concern is that of being able to satisfy his partner sexually, then size usually does not matter much. The most important component to a satisfying sexual life is the ability to satisfy one's partner.

In a heterosexual relationship, most women do not correlate the size of the penis with the probability of a partner being able to satisfy them sexually, although this is not always the case. For approximately 20% of women, size is important. And for another 1 % size is very important!

The majority of women are unable to achieve an orgasm through vaginal intercourse alone. However, for that group of women who do achieve vaginal orgasm, size may be of greater significance. The average stretched-length of the vagina is 3 to 4 inches, so for most partners the average penile length of 5 inches is more than accommodating. For years, the literature emphasized this point and reassured men that their average to below average-sized penis was all any woman needed to satisfy them. While that is often the case, for some women (i.e., size-obsessed Samantha from Sex in the City), that is absolutely not the case for others.

There clearly are women who could not care less about the size of the penis. Dr. Ernest Grafenberg (the famed-physician who first described the G spot) noted that there were innumerable erotogenic spots distributed all over the body from where sexual satisfaction can be elicited. He went on to say that almost no part of the female body does not give sexual response. The partner has only to find the erotogenic zones. So, while some women will only be fulfilled with a large penis, others will find satisfaction with stimulation of areas other than their vagina. Also, while men may focus more on the length of their penis, women actually prefer girth to length.

Penis size has symbolized masculinity, strength, endurance, ability, courage, intelligence, knowledge, all symbols of loving and being loved. Men with larger penises have a better body image. Statistically, men who rate themselves subjectively as having a larger penis tend to rate their own physical appearance higher. They also feel better about their sexual competence. There is a cultural influence suggesting a correlation between a large penis size and masculinity.

69% of all men view their penises as being average, 5% felt that they were larger than average and 26% felt that they were smaller than average. If a man knew how little importance most women place on penis size, this likely would result in the alleviation of the anxiety. The media is largely responsible for the dissemination of the belief that penis size is of paramount importance to most women. Popular literature would leave many men to believe that a six-inch erect penis is the norm. This is factually incorrect. In addition, while many women do find size to be very important, the majority of women do not.

SECTION 5

Penis Size Among Homosexuals

Men who identify themselves as homosexuals tend to have larger penises when compared with men who identify themselves as heterosexual. Furthermore, only 7% of men who identify themselves as being homosexual report a below average sized penis, which compares quite favorably compared to those in the heterosexual community. Penis size also influences the nature of the relationship in the homosexual community. Homosexuals with larger penises are more likely to identify themselves as tops or anal insertive. Those with smaller penises are more likely to be bottoms or anal-receptive.

SECTION 6

Size From A Woman's Perspective

Women are attracted to many different features of men, such as personality, kindness, warmth, attentiveness, shared-values, sense of humor, confidence, physical appearance and grooming. The Real Housewives of Beverly Hills find men with a big fat wallet very attractive. A physically fit guy may have an improved body image, which can affect self confidence, and a man with a large penis may reap similar benefits. At the end of the day, for most women, penis size is not at the top of the list. In fact, some women prefer no penis at all! (a.k.a. lesbians).

90% of women prefer a wide penis to a long penis. Most women, when asked, prioritize grooming over penis size. Women who have frequent vaginal orgasms climax more frequently with men with large penises. 33% of women prefer a longer than average size penis [a "size queen" is a popular slang term for a woman (or a man for that matter) who puts undue pressure on their partners to have a formidable-sized organ]. 60% stated that size made no difference and 6% felt large penises were less pleasurable.

That women favor larger penises has been confirmed in surveys of physical attractiveness of 3-dimensional images. The fact that men have larger penises both by comparison to other primates such as gorillas suggests a selection-bias in mating with men with larger penises. That means that historically, men with larger penises have been more successful in mating than men with smaller penises. This has resulted in a selection bias, which explains why men have relatively larger penises than other primates. Apparently, female gorillas are less discriminating than their human cohorts.

Why do women prefer girth over length?

Most women do not orgasm through vaginal penetration and many times it is only achieved through clitoral stimulation. The girth of the penis places the vagina on lateral stretch, and in that fashion the clitoris is brought closer to physical stimulation. Some researchers feel that the vagina is not constructed to achieve orgasm.

The G spot which is located in the lower third of the vagina, and the clitoris are the center for sexual stimulation. Only 30% of women reach orgasm during penile vaginal intercourse. 10 % to 15 % never climax under any circumstance.

The myth of deep vaginal penetration

The most sensitive part of the vagina is the part closest to the outside. This part is four inches deep. Most penises are easily able to stimulate this. With adequate stimulation, the vagina usually stretches or contracts to accommodate the penis, large or small.

For most women, stimulation of the deep vagina is not as important as the part of the vagina closest to the outside. However, as with most things sexual, not everyone is the same, and there clearly are those women who do crave deep stimulation. A partner with a smaller or even moderate-sized penis may not be able to satisfy that woman with vaginal intercourse alone. However, the G spot is located on the lower third of the vagina, where sensation is greatest, and the overwhelming majority of men are naturally built to adequately stimulate most women. That being said, not all women feel the same. There are women who will only be satisfied with a long, thick penis and a man with an average-sized penis will not be able to satisfy them with vaginal intercourse. This simple fact is NEVER discussed formally during any urology or gynecology residency and most doctors will not confirm this when asked.

SECTION 7

Is Bigger Better?

The short answer to this question is not always, but sometimes. In ancient Greece, a small penis was considered favorable. In ancient Greek art, smaller penises were actually glorified (statue of David!). Larger penises were attached to monsters like Satyr, and ugly old men. Satyr had horse-like features and a horse-sized penis which was constantly erect. He was a lecher and spent all of his time chasing nymphs. Satyr and his giant penis seemed to have a great time, but he was mocked, not glorified. Even now, not every man desires a large penis. In fact, 0.2% of men wish their penis was smaller!

While some women are more likely to orgasm with a larger penis, there is a group of women who prefer a smaller penis and find a smaller penis more pleasurable and less uncomfortable. In most surveys, partners prioritize rigidity over size. Some partners have been known to say "it's not the size of the wand, but the skill of the magician".

2

How Am I Doing?

The Disconnect Between Men And Women

45 % of men are not satisfied with the size of their penis, yet only 6 % of women feel their partner has a smaller than average-size penis. The explanation for this conundrum is simple; many men with average-size penises think that they are small compared to the average and, in fact, are not. Sometimes this can be corrected with education, but sometimes this alone is not enough. The media and popular culture are largely to blame.

Six inches is not the norm!!! Five inches is!!! In addition, in general, men seem to put much greater significance upon penis size than women do. Too many men are concerned that their penis may not be large enough to sexually satisfy their partner. The reality is that many women never achieve orgasm through penile vaginal intercourse no matter the size of the penis. The majority of women simply do not put much importance on penis size.

The Average-Sized Erect Penis Is Probably Smaller Than You Think!

There have been a number of studies about penis size. Interestingly, the results of the studies are quite variable. The studies can be categorized as scientific or surveys based upon personal observations. As one might expect, the studies based upon personal observations tend to reflect larger penises than those based upon actual scientific measurements. Who knew?

The average proximal measurement of girth was 4.7 inches closest to the abdominal wall and was 4.3 inches towards the tip proximal to the glans penis (a.k.a., the head). Heterosexual men focus on length. They actually should be more concerned about girth, which is most important to women. A wider penis promotes more clitoral stimulation, as the lateral stretching of the vagina draws the clitoris to physical stimulation. The clitoris is the center of sexual stimulation for most women.

The average flaccid length is between 3.5 and 3.8 inches long. Again, there is very little correlation between the size of a flaccid penis and the size of an erect penis. Penises grow between .5 and 3.5 inches when erect. Smaller penises tend to grow more than large penises. In fact, smaller penises tend to grow up to 50% more then large penises when erect. In layman's terms, there are showers (a person who has a large, flaccid penis with limited growth upon erection) and growers (those who have a flaccid penis that grows significantly when stimulated). Most surgical interventions, in fact, affect the flaccid length more than the erect length.

The average stretched penis length is 5 1/4 inches. 55% of men have erect penises of 5.5 inches or less. Any penis greater than 3.66 inches falls within the 2.5 standard deviation of normal. 95% of penises are between 4.2 and 7.5 inches.

Where does the myth of the 6 inch penis come from? The Kinsey Report is one of the most famous studies of sex ever performed. In 1948, Kinsey questioned 3,500 college men and asked them to self-measure their stretched penile length. This is self reported. Do men ever lie about the size of their penis? Hell yes! Studies in which investigators measure the size of penis tend to be 1 inch less than studies in which an individual is asked to measure his own genitalia.

So the upshot is that studies in which length is determined by impartial observers (and not self-reported) indicate that the average stretched penis length (which closely approximates erect length) is 5 inches.

SECTION 3

See Yourself As Others See You, Not As You See You

One of the reasons that approximately 50% of all men are concerned about the size of their penis is because their perspective may be distorted. Most guys look at their penis from above, which will naturally make it look smaller.

When men look at other men in the locker room, they're looking at a penis with a different perspective. They're looking at a penis from the side or from in front. This makes the other penises look bigger! It may be helpful to look at yourself in front of a full length mirror naked to get a different perspective. Of course, this seems so simple, but it really seems to make a difference. You may be bigger than you think.

SECTION 4

How To Measure Your Penis

One can measure the penis in either the flaccid or the erect state. These measurements will obviously be quite different.

There is very little correlation between the size of the flaccid penis and the erect penis. In fact, men can be split into two categories, showers and growers. Men who have smaller flaccid penises tend to grow relatively more than men with larger flaccid penises.

Other factors besides erection that can influence the measured size of the penis include the frequency of sexual intercourse and the temperature. Cold temperatures can cause the penis to temporarily shrink (as noted by George in the famous "shrinkage" Seinfeld episode where George goes for a swim in the ocean, penis shrinkage occurs and a woman sees it, resulting in his great humiliation). Physiologically, the reason that the penis shrinks with cold temperature is because of a contraction of the dartos muscle.

Measuring Length

The most useful measurement of length is SPL, which is stretched penile length. This is the measurement which correlates best with erect length. The penis rests in front of the pubic bone. One places the end of the ruler on top of the penis against the pubic bone. The stretched penis length is the measurement from the bone to the tip of the penis. This measurement is performed while stretching the penis. This is also referred to as the bone-pressed length, as you are literally pressing against the pubic bone during this measurement. Measuring the penis in this manner will pleasantly surprise many guys.

As we get older, we tend to gain weight centrally. As a consequence, many men feel that their penis is shrinking when in fact it is the fat surrounding the penis which is increasing. A lot of men have small penises in the resting state (flaccid) that actually grow significantly when stimulated. As previously stated, these men are called growers. Measuring the stretched penis length will help to clarify their actual length.

Measuring girth

The most useful measurements for girth are obtained with a full erection. Some simply measure the girth at its widest point. Others utilize a tape measure at the base of the penis, and a second measurement of the circumference is obtained towards the tip of the penis, proximal to the glans or head of the penis. Most men have more girth at the base of the penis than at the end of the shaft near the glans. If performing penis stretching exercises, in order to track growth, always try to measure at the same spot.

SECTION 5

Penile Girth

While most men focus on the length of their penis, women actually find girth more important sexually. In fact 90% of women prefer a wide penis to a long one. In order to measure the girth, one should use a vinyl measuring tape. As an alternative you could use a string and a ruler.

The most important measure of girth is determined with an erect penis. Without an erection, the girth will depend upon one's emotional state or the temperature. The girth should be obtained at its widest point. The average erect girth is 4.7 to 5.1 inches.

Procedures designed to increase penis size are more successful changing the girth then they are the length. All of the girth-enhancing fillers are placed between dartos fascia and Buck's fascia. The rate-limiting step in terms of enhancing the girth is a function of how far the delicate overlying skin and fascia can be stretched. Too much pressure will result in necrosis (permanent death of cell tissue) of the skin.

Any material used to increase girth should be long-acting or absorbed slowly and uniformly. If the material is absorbed in an irregular fashion, this will result in a lumpy, deformed penis. A guiding principle in plastic surgery is to replace like with like. The more the material is similar to natural tissue, the better the results.

SECTION 6

Is It All In Your Head?

Small penis syndrome can be part of body dysmorphobia (also known as body dysmorphic disorder). This is a fixation on an imaginary flaw in physical appearance. Taken to an extreme, patients with this disorder can become depressed or suicidal. Some patients with this disorder avoid social situations and intimate relationships. Also, some with this disorder feel that they have to change the affected body part in order to reach any type of happiness.

There are an estimated 200,000 cases per year in United States of BDD (Body Dysmorphic Disorder). It can't be cured but can be treated. The "flaw" may be minor or imagined but the person spends hours a day trying to fix it. These patients tend to be young and perfectionists. They may be narcissists. Patients may try cosmetic procedures or exercise to excess. People with this condition constantly compare their appearance with that of others. Treatment could mean counseling and antidepressant medication. Associated moods include anxiety, general discontent, compulsive behavior and depression. It has also been called imagined ugliness.

Some think that imbalances in neurotransmitters such as serotonin may have a role in body dysmorphia. Others feel it's a consequence of our image-obsessed culture. It could be biochemical or a consequence of external forces of our culture.

Small penis syndrome is characterized by men who have a normal-sized penis but are anxious about the size of their penis. This category probably fits a substantial portion of all men. Small penis syndrome is different than micropenis, which is a condition characterized by an anatomically abnormally small penis. Generally, a micropenis is considered less than 2.75 inches long when erect. Only about 0.6% (or 1 in 200) of all men suffer from micropenis.

Some other psychiatric disorders may encourage over-preoccupation with the size of a patient's genitalia. Narcissism involves infatuation and obsession with an individual excluding concern for other people.

If a patient has a normal-sized penis and is still over-preoccupied, this can result in abnormal social behavior. Some may avoid certain types of social situations, avoid public restrooms and avoid certain work situations because of irrational concerns about their penis size. Some of these patients may benefit from psychological or psychiatric intervention.

A man with a normal sized penis having some insecurities is common and not pathological. When these insecurities are taken to an extreme form and influence social behavior that may fall into the category of a psychiatric disorder. On the other hand, many people who are completely healthy psychologically have a desire to enhance their physical appearance. If improving one's physical appearance results in a generalized sense of well-being or greater confidence, this is to be encouraged as long as one can do so in a safe manner.

As with any medical treatment, patients have an absolute right to make an informed decision about their health care. This decision must be one based on realism. It is incumbent upon providers not to prey upon patients whose decisions may be clouded by unrealistic expectations. Just as some men who are completely well adjusted choose to spend hours in the gym weightlifting to improve their physical appearance and feel better about themselves, some men have a strong desire to have a larger penis.

While it is commonly accepted that some women want to undergo surgery to enhance the size of their breasts, there is no such similar widespread acceptance of men wishing to increase the size of their penis. As the methods and techniques of penile enhancement continue to evolve, acceptance is likely to become more widespread.

SECTION 7

Terms That Sound Similar But Are Very Different: PDS

Penile Dysmorphic Syndrome (a.k.a. Penile Dysmorphophobia) or small penis syndrome: This is an extremely common condition which involves a high percentage of all men. Far more men feel that their penis is smaller than average compared to men who think that their penis is larger than average. There is a huge disconnect between the realities of a bell-shaped curve and men's own perception of where they fall on the curve.

Common reasons for this condition include the fact that men usually examine the size of their own penis looking down rather than looking at a full length mirror. It also doesn't help that the only other men commonly seen with an erection are those who are porn stars. Education alone can commonly cure this condition. The average erect penis size is 5 inches, not 6 inches!

Inconspicuous Penis Or Buried Penis

Men tend to gain weight with an uneven distribution. Typically, men tend to gain weight in their waist, and in particular, the area surrounding their penis. Thus, many men with a normal-sized penis appear to have a much smaller phallus than is actually the case, simply because the penis is buried in surrounding fat. It is commonly stated that a loss of 35 pounds of weight may result in an apparent gain of 1 inch of penile length. Liposuction of the fat surrounding the penis is one of the strategies employed by penis enhancement surgeons. This can serve a dual purpose as the lipoaspirate can also be used to enhance the penile girth with free fat transfer.

Micropenis

Fortunately, true micropenis is quite rare with approximately 0.6% of all men being so afflicted (about 1 in 200 men). By definition, a micropenis is 2.5 standard deviation's less than the mean penile length. Most urologists recognize a stretched penis length of 2.75 inches as a micropenis. Congenital micropenis is likely a consequence of inadequate testosterone production during the second and third trimester.

Other potential causes can include a failure of tissues to respond to available testosterone. A neonate with a penis less than .75 inches is considered to have micropenis. Even though inadequate testosterone production during gestation is the cause, giving additional testosterone to an adult is not the answer. Testosterone supplementation after puberty has little influence on penile size.

Webbed Penis

A webbed penis is a normal length penis which appears to be shorter than its actual length because of a web of tissue connecting the penis to the scrotum. This is largely a cosmetic issue. This can easily be corrected with a relatively minor surgical procedure.

A webbed scrotum does not actually interfere with the erect length of the penis. This does not affect the stretched penile length, measuring from the pubic bone to the tip of the penis. However, looking at the penis laterally (from the side), the junction of the penis and scrotum is closer to mid-shaft, rather than at the base. Removing the web moves this junction back closer to the base.

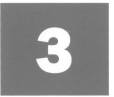

Anatomy and Physiology

Examination Of The Penis

The penis should be examined in both the flaccid as well as erect state. The angle of the erection varies dependent upon the size of the penis and the looseness of the suspensory ligament. Larger penises tend to hang lower and may not achieve an erection greater than 90°. Smaller penises tend to point nearly straight up.

Some penises bend to the right or to the left. One of the common conditions that cause this is Peyronie's disease. In Peyronie's disease, one or more plaques are formed on the tunica albuginea of the corpora cavernosa. A plaque is fibrotic tissue, like gristle. It is a type of connective tissue disorder. As a consequence of the plaque, the corpora cannot expand normally. This results in a bent phallus with erections. It can cause penile folding and pain with erections. It can also be a cause of erectile dysfunction. Up to 8% or more of all men will experience Peyronie's disease in their lifetime. The prevalence of Peyronie's disease is 3.2%.

Another common cause of penises that are bent with erection is corporal disproportion, where the two corpora are of different lengths. This can cause the penis to bend to the right or to the left. If the penis naturally bends down, the two corpora may be disproportionate to the underlying urethra. These are congenital conditions, whereas Peyronie's disease is acquired. In other words, patients who have corporal disproportion are born with the condition and have this condition their entire lives.

Patients with Peyronie's disease initially have a straight penis with erection that changes later in life. Peyronie's disease is most common between the ages of 40 and 60. Some people believe that Peyronie's disease is caused by the trauma of sexual intercourse, where microtears are produced in the tunica albuginea and later calcify. This can occur during intercourse, when you zig when you should have zagged. For other patients, it may be a type of autoimmune disease, as patients with Dupytren's contracture (a somewhat similar condition that affects the hand) have a higher propensity to developing Peyronie's disease. The plaques can cause the size of the erect penis to decrease over time. The plaques can sometimes be treated with an injectable enzyme or Verapamil, which helps to dissolve plaque. Other surgeons try to cut the plaques out and graft the subsequent defects created in the tunica.

Patients who are uncircumcised should be able to freely move the foreskin over the glans penis. If the foreskin is stuck over the glans this is called phimosis, and if it is stuck before the glans penis, this is called paraphimosis.

The urethral orifice is typically located at the tip of the glans penis. During development, some patients develop a urethral orifice at an atypical position such as the proximal glans or the end of the shaft. This condition is called hypospadias, and is usually corrected in childhood. Patients who have hypospadias may have an abnormal shape to their glans.

Almost every systemic rash that can occur anywhere on the body may also appear on the penis. Common general skin conditions that can also occur on the penis include psoriasis, eczema and allergy dermatitis. In addition, many sexually transmitted diseases will first become evident on the penis. Any type of urethral discharge, or the appearance of blood at the urethral orifice or in the urine, is a warning sign requiring medical attention.

Cancer of the penis is quite rare and usually only occurs in uncircumcised men. Vitiligo is a common condition which results in a loss of pigmentation on patches of the skin. Certainly any new rashes of the penis should prompt one to seek rapid medical attention. The development of a new bend in the erect penis should also prompt one to be evaluated by a physician.

SECTION 2

Anatomy Of The Penis

The corpora cavernosa are two large cylinders that are responsible for producing an erection. The corpora cavernosa reside on the dorsum (top) of the penis. The vital nerves responsible for sensation of the penis rest

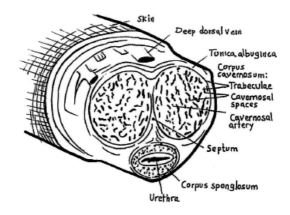

on top of the corpora cavernosa. On the bottom of the penis resides the corpus spongiosum which contains the urethra responsible for transport of urine.

The glans penis, or head of the penis is an expansion of the corpus spongiosum distally.

Approximately one-half of the penis resides inside of the body. In other words, one can only visibly see one half of the penis. The two large cylinders responsible for erections, the corpora cavernosa, reside under the pubis. The superficial fundiform ligament (also called the falciform ligament) and the deeper suspensory ligament (also called the triangular or arcuate ligament) attach the penis under the pubis. Cutting the suspensory ligament is one of the mainstays of penile-lengthening surgery, allowing part of the internal penis to come out.

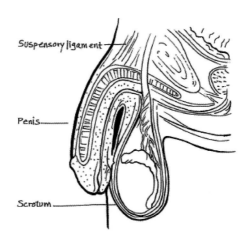

The penis is surrounded by pre pubic fat. As the amount of pre-pubic fat increases this can result in the appearance of a smaller penis. Removing this pre-pubic fat by either diet and/or exercise or with liposuction will give one the appearance of a larger penis.

Some patients suffer from a hidden penis which is a condition characterized by a normal-sized penis enveloped in fat. A hidden penis will have a diminished flaccid length, but a normal stretched penile length, which is determined by measuring from the pubic bone to the tip of the penis.

Buck's fascia is a thick protective layer that covers the corpora cavernosa and splits to surround the urethra. The various bulking agents which include free fat, hyaluronic acid derivatives, alloderm, and others are all placed between the skin and Buck's fascia. Dartos fascia is loosely attached to Buck's fascia, so it is relatively easy to place either a sheet of tissue or various liquid forms between the two layers. The bulking agents are generally placed on top of the corpora cavernosa and not under the corpus spongiosum to avoid injuring the urethra.

SECTION 3

How The Penis Works

"The penis does not obey the order of its master, who tries to erect or shrink it at will. Instead, the penis erects freely while its master is asleep. The penis must be said to have its own mind, by any stretch of the imagination." Leonardo da Vinci.

Historically, a number of incorrect theories were held to rationalize the kinetics of erections. Aristotle thought that erections were due to an influx of air. In 1585, Pare correctly identified an erection as the product of increased blood-flow to the penis. "When the man becomes inflamed with lust and desire blood rushes into the male member and causes it to become erect."

Even when the penis is flaccid (in a relaxed state) the length varies. This is a function of one's emotional state as well as the temperature. This is controlled by smooth muscle in the penis.

The most important feature of a penis in sexual intercourse is rigidity. This is dependent upon the amount of blood flowing into the penis as well as penile geometry. A penis that is bent downwards will have a greater challenge staying rigid during intercourse. This is a very important point in penile enlargement surgery. The penis is secured under the pubic bone by the suspensory ligament. One of the most common procedures performed for the purposes of enlargement is ligamentolysis, or division of the suspensory ligament. The suspensory ligament does prevent the internal penis from being pulled out.

About one half of your penis is naturally inside of your body. While many men would like to pull this part of the penis out to give them more length, by doing so there is a loss of some support. Losing this support changes the geometry of the penis. Although the operation should not impair the blood flow to the penis, there may be a downward deflection, which may make sexual intercourse more challenging.

The corpora cavernosa are the two large cylinders in the penis that create most of the rigidity of an erection. The corpora are covered by the tunica albuginea, which is very durable and strong. This thick cover is what allows the blood in the corpora cavernosa to become so rigid during an erection. The corpora cavernosa run part way into the glans penis or head of the penis. The tip of the penis is composed of corpus spongiosum which does not contain a capsule like the tunica albuginea. It really serves as a soft cushion to prevent injury to the inner vagina and cervix.

There are smooth muscles in the corpora cavernosa and lining the arteries. When the penis is flaccid the smooth muscles are contracted. When the weather is cold the muscles contract even more. This results in less blood flowing into the penis. The contraction of the smooth muscles in the corpora and arteries is the reason poor George experienced the infamous shrinkage after coming out of the ocean on Seinfeld!

Biochemistry Of An Erection

With sexual stimulation, there is a release of neurotransmitters, such as nitric oxide. This causes the smooth muscle in the arteries and corpora cavernosa to relax, which causes an increase in blood flow into the penis. When the corpora cavernosa expand, this actually closes off the veins by compression, so there is a net increase of blood in, and decrease of blood out.

The angle of the erection is dependent upon the size of the penis and it's suspension to the pubic bone. Men with longer, heavier penises have a looser attachment to the pubic bone and have a less acute angle of erection. In men with larger penises, they may not achieve an angle of greater than 90° with a full erection. Larger penises hang lower and don't angle as much up.

As mentioned earlier, there is no thick capsule in the glans as there is in the shaft. The head of the penis only becomes one third as rigid as the shaft. The glans does not trap blood as efficiently as the shaft does.

On a biochemical level, the release of nitric oxide stimulates the production of cGMP, which opens and closes potassium channels. This, in turn, relaxes the smooth muscle resulting in an increase in blood flow to the penis. Pills such as Viagra prevent the degradation of cGMP by inhibiting PDE5. This results in continued relaxation of the smooth muscle, and, hence, continued blood flow into the penis.

SECTION 4

Medical Conditions May Cause The Penis To Shrink

There are several medical conditions which can result in shortening of the penis. A condition known as Peyronie's disease affects approximately 8% of all men over their lifetime, making this one of the most common urological conditions. Peyronie's disease results in the creation of plaques on the corpora cavernosa. The corpora are the two cylinder-like structures in the penis which fill with blood resulting in erection. Patients who suffer from this condition develop a penis which is crooked or bent when erect. These patients may have pain when they are erect. This also results in a foreshortening of the penis, as a crooked penis has less effective length.

Radical prostatectomy for the treatment of prostate cancer frequently results in subsequent shortening of the penis. Some patients lose up to 15% of their penile length following surgery. Up to 48% of men undergoing this form of surgery experience shortening greater than 1.0 cm. Connecting the urethra to the neck of the bladder may result in a telescoping type of effect resulting in shortening of the penis. Some investigators feel that the shortening of the penis after prostatectomy may be a consequence of the subsequent development of erectile dysfunction in some patients. Because of this frequent outcome of reduced penile length following surgery, some have advocated the routine use of vacuum erection devices following this form of treatment.

It is commonly believed that prolonged periods of sexual inactivity, particularly in men who do not have nocturnal erections may also result in shortening of the penis. In fact, objective studies confirm that patients who suffer from erectile dysfunction do have comparatively smaller penises. It may be that when men have erections there is an increase in blood flow to the penis and this is beneficial in reference to maintaining size. One way to think of this is that every time a man has an erection, he is exercising his penis.

Even when men are not sexually active they have nocturnal erections. When men become impotent they stop having spontaneous erections at night when they are asleep. Men who suffer from impotency stop having the nocturnal erections and put themselves at risk for a decline in the size of their phallus. Patients who undergo a combination of androgen deprivation in conjunction with radiation therapy have been shown to have decreased penile size.

SECTION 5

Relevant Female Anatomy

It is estimated up to 40 % of women have a complaint of sexual dysfunction. Up to 63% of women have arousal or orgasmic dysfunction. Women report the strongest orgasm and least effort to achieve an orgasm with stimulation of the area above the clitoris. They report less sexual sensitivity for the vagina than for the external genitalia.

The greatest nerve density is above and fanning out from the clitoris. The area superior to them (directly over the clitoris) is the most sensitive. The maximum nerve density is in those areas. That is why most women do not achieve orgasm through vaginal intercourse alone.

The clitoris, urethra, and end of the vagina together form a type of unified entity.

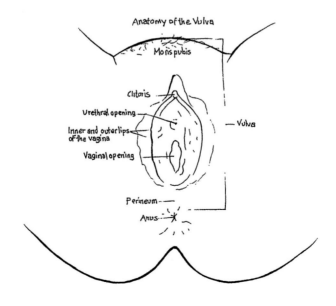

They have a shared nerve supply and blood supply.

Two thirds of women reported a longer penis either made no difference in their likelihood of reaching orgasm or made it less likely they would climax. One third of women indicated that longer penises and deep penetration were more helpful for achieving orgasm. Some women do desire deep penetration which reaches the cervix. In other words, some women are able to reach orgasm through cervical stimulation.

Since the vagina is 3 to 7 inches long there may be some women who can only achieve orgasm with a longer penis. For most women, that is not the case. A woman with a long vagina who can only achieve orgasm through cervical stimulation may not be able to achieve an orgasm with vaginal intercourse with a man with a shorter penis. This could result in a mismatch. So, there is no hard and fast rule.

Some women will only be satisfied with a partner with a large penis and for others this is absolutely not true. But even for guys that are size-challenged, it is likely that they would be able to satisfy their partners with a little creativity.

CHAPTER

4 | **Penis Enlargement Supplements**

SECTION 1

Herbal Medicine

Herbal medicine is now recognized as offering potential significant benefits in a host of medical challenges. There are herbal medicine departments at top medical centers including Harvard and UCLA (incorporated into integrative medicine). According to the World Health Organization, 80% of all people use some form of herbal remedies in their healthcare. Approximately 25 % of Americans who see a physician about a health problem are already using some form of unconventional therapy.

There are virtually an infinite number of products sold on the market which espouse their ability to enlarge a client's penis. Herbal supplements are not subject to the same rigorous testing as are prescription drugs approved by the FDA. There is some regulation in terms of assuring that the products are pure and produced in a sanitary environment.

While no pill alone is likely to result in a substantial increase in penis size, some supplements may offer benefits when combined with penis stretching, exercises or surgery. These treatments could be thought of as complementary or something done along with recognized treatment.

There is a misheld belief that "natural" supplements are always safe and have no health risks. Unfortunately, that is not universally true. Even herbal supplements, when taken in extreme amounts, can be dangerous. In addition, some supplements adversely react with prescription medication. Always consult with your personal physician when taking medication. Included is a description of some of the common elements that are found in penis supplements. Many of the products have a theoretical benefit in increasing blood flow, and perhaps affecting the production of sex hormones. That does not necessarily translate into penis enlargement.

The addition of testosterone after puberty has not been shown to increase penis size (if testosterone did increase penis size there would be an explosion in the testosterone replacement marketplace). If the addition of testosterone after puberty does not affect penis size, there is no rationale for the use of products that supposedly help to increase testosterone levels.

Testosterone does have a role in sexual function and sexual desire. It has a role in physical performance, strength and lean body mass. Similarly, increasing blood flow may have beneficial affects on the quality of an erection, but is unlikely to affect the size of a man's phallus.

Traction therapy has been shown to increase length by cell division and cell growth. As such, supplements that support this process on a cellular level may be beneficial. Cell growth requires an increase in cytoplasmic and organelle volume with an increase in genetic material. Cell division requires the parent cell to divide into two or more daughter cells. Supplements that support the process of cell growth and cell division and the production of collagen may prove to be particularly beneficial to augment the affects of traction therapy as well as injection treatments.

Listed below are some of the common components found in contemporary penis enlargement products. In addition are listed some of the newer components which may actually promote collagen production, cell growth and cell division.

SECTION 2

Common Components Of Penis Enlargement Pills

Antioxidants. Antioxidant nutrients include vitamin A C, E, and selenium. These can be part of a supplement or can be obtained by eating fruits vegetables beans and whole grains. Most of us should all be eating a minimum of five servings of fruits and vegetables every day.

Antioxidants help with the circulation and increased blood flow in general. Vitamin D is manufactured by the body when exposed to sunlight. It is involved in the production of hormones, and enzymes, and growth factors. Vitamin E is found in fresh green vegetables, meat, egg yolks. It can repair damage caused by free radicals. Vitamin C can help reduce cholesterol and it is present in oranges and berries. Vitamin C helps the body produce collagen.

Astragalus Membranaceus. Overall health benefits include a possible assist to the immune system.

Avena Sativa. It is also known as oat straw, or the common oat. It may increase sexual desire and performance.

Butea Superba. It is a vine that grows in India, China, Vietnam and Thailand. It is reported to increase sexual performance. It may possibly have an effect on hormone levels. Not well studied in humans, erection studies have been performed on rats.

Caltrop. It enhances hormone levels. It is also reported to improve energy and vitality.

Citrulline. It is a ubiquitous amino acid in mammals, related to arginine and has been shown to increase erection hardness.   It is a precursor to NO.

Ginkgo Biloba. It blocks a platelet-activating factor, giving it a blood thinning effect. As might be expected, one of the side effects is bleeding. It can react adversely with other blood thinning agents such as Coumadin, aspirin, or persantine. It is an antioxidant preventing the damage caused by free radicals. It may relax vascular smooth muscle and in that fashion increase blood flow. Ginkgo Biloba may improve circulation. It has been found to be somewhat effective in treating erectile dysfunction in patients with depression.

Herbs Cistanches. It is reportedly beneficial for sexual health. It has antioxidant, neuroprotective and anti-aging qualities. It also may help kidney disease.

Horny Goat Weed. It is known to increase testosterone in animals. The active ingredient is Icarlin, which may promote erections. It works by relaxing smooth muscle. It has been reported to contribute an anti-aging effect. Excessive doses can cause dizziness, vomiting, bleeding from the nose.

L Arginine. L Arginine is a precursor of nitric oxide (NO). NO is a neuro transmitter responsible for dilation of blood vessels and is an important component of the erection cascade. L Arginine has been shown to increase blood circulation. It has been shown to stimulate the release of growth hormone. It also may reduce the risk of stroke and blood clots. Human trials regarding the use of L Arginine in patients with erectile dysfunction have yielded mixed results. It seems to have its greatest effect on patients with vascular disease.

Licorice Root. It may prevent the breakdown of adrenal hormones. It also may have an effect on reduction of plaques in blood vessels. There is a potential adverse interaction with Warfarin (a blood thinner).

Maca Powder. This is an anti-oxidant that may boost energy as well as the immune system. It is a root found in the Peruvian Andes and belongs to the mustard family. It has amino acids, iron, iodine and magnesium. There is very limited human data to confirm its effect on sexual performance.

Niacin (VitaminB3). It is important for the production of the sex hormones including testosterone. It increases the production of prostaglandins. It also helps to release histamine and has a role in the dilation of blood vessels, particularly small capillaries such as those that serve the penis. It may enhance cell metabolism and increase absorption of carbohydrates. It may cause flushing.

Panax Ginseng. It may increase the production of nitric oxide and may also act as an antioxidant. It may also increase penile rigidity. Overall, the mechanism of action is not clear, and most prospective studies have not been convincing.

Pumpkin Seeds. It has free radical scavenging antioxidants. It is high in magnesium, which is involved in the synthesis of RNA and DNA, high in Zinc and may support prostate health.

Propionyl-L-Carnitine. It is an amino acid produced by the body. Amino acids are the building blocks of proteins. It is sometimes used in conjunction with acetyl L carnitine to try to increase testerone levels. It may help to increase circulation. It also has anti-oxidant properties. It is well tolerated and has few side effects.

Pycnogenol. It helps to boost the synthesis of nitric oxide along with L Arginine. There is insufficient evidence to rate for effectiveness for treatment of erectile dysfunction. It is an extract of French maritime pine bark and serves as a scavanger of free radicals. It has demonstrated anti-inflammatory activity in animals. It also dilates small blood vessels.

Pyridoxine (Vitamin B6). It is important in the formation of red blood cells and important for many bodily functions. It has a role in the formation of male sex hormones. It also has a role in the production of neurotransmitters. It may help to increase the response to sexual stimulation. It is present in yeast, liver, eggs, milk, salmon, avocados and vegetables. Additionally, it is a component of many body building regimens. Although water soluble vitamins are generally considered safe, high doses of pyridoxine have been associated with sensory neuropathy.

Rhizoma Cucurmae Longae. It affects blood flow.

Rhodiola Rosea. It may increase erectile function.

Saw Palmetto. It supports prostate health. Studies indicate favorable outcomes when compared to other products such as Finasteride (used to treat symptoms of an enlarged prostate).

Stinging Nettle Root. It may address prostate conditions, is a low level diuretic and may decrease inflammation. This is not well studied.

Tongkat Ali. It has been reported to benefit premature ejaculation. It has aphrodisiac, antimicrobial and anti-pyretic activities.

Tribulus Terrestris. It Improves erections perhaps by increasing DHEA levels, specifically, protodioscin. It is also referred to as Libilov, which is a phytochemical derived from the Tribulus Terrestris plant and is converted to DHEA and, thus, presumably has a beneficial sexual effect. These claims are largely unproven in the human model, studies were done on rats. It is felt that DHEA is required for maintenance of cell membrane integrity.

Tricopus Zeylanicus. It is derived from a plant from India. This product is used to increase sex drive. The mechanism of action is unknown.

Velvet Deer Antler. It is reported to contain a substance similar to IGF1 (insulin-like growth factor). It is thought to stimulate growth in muscle tissue. IGF1 has anabolic effects in adults. It has been shown to increase strength and muscular endurance when combined with exercise by increased protein synthesis. It does not influence testosterone production.

Vitus Vinifera. It is also known as the common grapevine. This is native to the Mediterranean, Morocco and Iran. Fractions of the grape seeds are antioxidant rich. Grape skins contain Anthocyanins, which protects the connective tissue from degradation and improve circulation.

Xanthoparmelia Scabrosa. It is made up of algae and fungus living together. It is reported to increase sexual performance and desire.

Yohimbine. One of the most frequently studied supplements for the treatment of erectile dysfunction. It has been found to be modestly effective in the treatment of erectile dysfunction. It may increase blood flow during erections. It is a central nervous system stimulant and an alpha 2 adranergic receptor antagonist. Yohimbine may cause headaches and raise blood pressure. It can elevate the heart rate. It can also cause agitation and sleeplessness.

Zinc. It serves as an important role in male sexual function and needed for production of testosterone. Zinc can be found in many natural foods such as beef, oysters, turkey and beans. It has a role in protein synthesis and cellular growth. Excessive amounts can result in an impaired immune system.

SECTION 3

Supplements Which May Promote Cell Division, Cell Growth, And Collagen Production:

Collagen Hydrolysate. It is high in Glycine, Lysine and Proline and may help promote cell growth and build connective tissue. It is also well absorbed, and has been found to have an excellent safety profile.

Collagen Peptide. It is a molecule of two or more amino acids. Collagen peptides have been used in the bodybuilding community to support muscle mass. Peptides contain 50 or less amino acids and are smaller than proteins. Hydrolyzed gelatin products have been designated as GRAS by the FDA (generally recognized as safe). Collagen peptide is well digested and well tolerated.

L Tyrosine. It supports cell growth and is a building block of protein. It is found in dairy, meat and fish, may raise thyroid hormone production and may interfere with absorption of certain medications.

L Glutamine. It supports protein synthesis and is the most abundant-free amino acid in the body. It also helps to provide nitrogen and carbon. It should be used with caution in patients with liver disease and those with a history of seizure disorder.

L Lysine. It is a precursor for other amino acids and crucial to the formation of collagen. It is also an essential amino acid that the body cannot produce. It is found in meat, cheese, fish, eggs and soy.

Methionine. It supports cell division and replication. It supplies sulfur, which is required for growth. Methionine is found in almonds, broccoli, beans, eggs, and fish.

Proline. It is a nonessential amino acid that the body can produce from other substrates.

Threonine. It is an amino acid also present in lentils, peanuts, eggs, beef and chicken. Threonine helps create glycine and serine, needed for the production of collagen and muscle tissue. Excess threonine may be hepatotoxic.

CHAPTER

5 | Penis Exercises

Stretching The Penis, Also Known As Penile Traction Therapy

Advocates of penis stretching hope for the lengthening of tissue through traction. The theory depends upon the production of microtears in the tissues of the penis with subsequent cellular growth and enlargement. It is postulated that this is a consequence of hyperplasia and cell division (cellular growth and replication). Basically, the traction forces the cells to spread further apart. The body reacts to this by creating new cells and larger cells.

Stretching can be accomplished in a number of different ways, which can vary from techniques as simple as pulling or stretching of the penis with one's hand versus elaborate mechanical tools, which extend the penis or facilitate hanging of weights from the penis. There is some evidence to suggest that these techniques may be helpful in achieving transient lengthening of the penis, and some reports have made claims regarding change in girth as well.

As with almost any form of intervention, there are always some risks. Taken to an extreme form, even stretching of the penis can result in damage to vital structures of the penis, including nerves and blood vessels.

Animal experiments have actually shown that the epidermis does respond to constant tension by increasing cell division. Animal experiments have also demonstrated that wounds subjected to stretching have increased numbers of myofibroblasts. These are involved in formation of the extracellular matrix and in the repair process. In simplified terms, they are the glue that forms a network of cells.

One might reasonably ask if constant stretching of body tissues has ever been shown to actually work. The concept does have validity and is actually applied in other forms of cosmetic surgery.

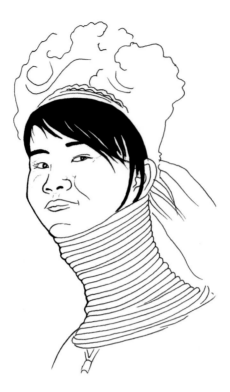

The use of temporary implants is well documented in plastic surgery. Plastic surgeons may temporarily use an implant to stretch the skin to facilitate subsequent tension-free closure when there is a lack of available skin. Orthopedic surgeons commonly use traction to try to stretch bones.

The Padaung tribe of Myanmar place metal coils around the necks of their females to successfully produce long necks in their females (who have been labeled giraffe women)!

In New Guinea, some tribes hang weights from the penises of children to try to achieve greater length. Advocates of stretching state that there should not be any pain when performing this exercise.

Hand stretching

Advocates of hand stretching of the penis referred to this as exercise for the penis and postulate that there may be an increase in smooth muscle of the penis with exercise. Some feel that there may be an increase in both length and girth with penis stretching. As with most forms of exercise, results tend to be slow and gradual. Some men have reported gains as great as 2 inches after one year of stretching. Even those fortunate men who did achieve this had great patience and perseverance.

Prior to initiating a period of stretching, it is advised that the phallus be warmed with either a wet towel or a sock filled with warm rice. Obviously, be careful that the rice in the sock is not too hot or you can burn your penis. One can fill half of a sock with rice and place it in a microwave along with a separate cup of water to humidify the rice. This should be warmed to a comfortable point.

Another way to warm up prior to initiating a session of stretching is to soak in a hot tub or take a warm shower. The advantage of the rice sock is that it allows you to keep the penis warm between exercises. The penis should be warm for 10 to 15 minutes prior to starting the session. The penis should also generally be semi-erect when starting the stretching session. Practitioners advise against a full erection. Stretching should be performed in a gentle, steady and slow fashion. Stretching can be done in a sitting or standing position.

Hand stretching involves placing one hand across the shaft of the penis and pulling the penis up, down and to the sides for 30 second intervals. One hand is placed 1 inch below the glans penis.

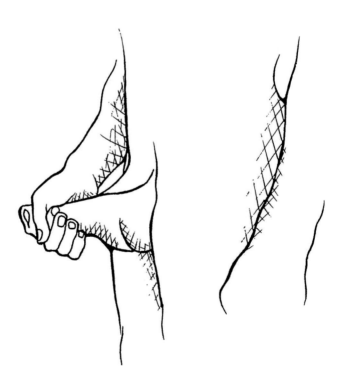

Never pull on the glans during these exercises, as it is much more delicate than the shaft. The stretching is never performed with a full erection. If the gentleman feels any pain, he should stop immediately. The other hand is used to place mild pressure on the perineum. The perineum is the area between the anus and the scrotum (in layman's terms, the taint!). With gentle steady pressure the penis is pulled out, up, down, to the right, and to the left.

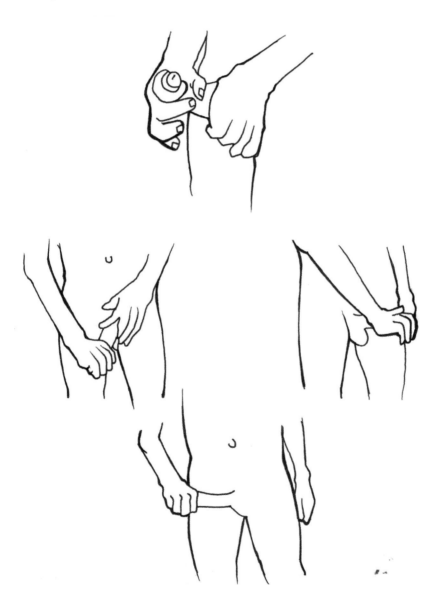

Each stretch is for 30 seconds, so to stretch in all five positions should take 150 seconds per set. Stretching is usually done in 2 sets for a total of 5 minutes. This should be done after the penis is warmed up. Stretching can then be followed by jelqing. Stretching is performed without lubrication, which is subsequently applied for the jelqing session (see Chapter 5, section 3).

In addition, the penis can be stretched by rotating the penis like a crank. One generally uses one hand for these stretching exercises, although additional pressure can be applied by removing the fingers from the perineum and placing the second hand on the penis during these stretching motions.

There are many different variations available for stretching. These can include lifting the leg, grasping the penis by placing the hand under the leg and then pulling on the penis towards the anus.

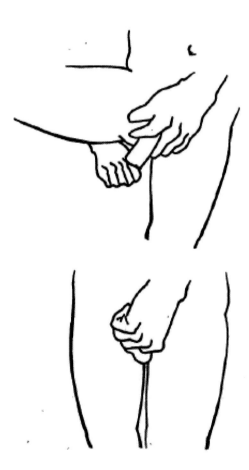

Another variation of stretching the penis employs traction and countertraction to specific zones of the penis. One hand is placed proximal to the glans penis and pulls the penis out while the second hand places pressure at the mid-shaft and pulls in, providing counter traction. Then, the second hand is placed at the base of the penis for an additional stretch. This would seem to involve sequential stretching of different parts of the penis.

Another described technique involves placing the OK-grip proximal to the glans penis and then resting the bottom surface of the penis on the contralateral wrist.

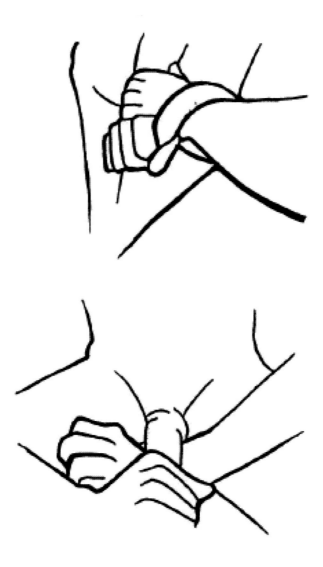

The penis is stretched over the wrist for a period of 10 seconds. Additional pressure can be obtained by grasping the contralateral arm with the free hand.

Yet another technique involves pulling the penis straight out with one hand placed in an overhand grip towards the end of the shaft. The webbing between the thumb and index finger of the second hand is then placed on the dorsal surface of the penis, and is pushed downward. This results in the penis assuming a V shape. By placing the V in different areas of the penis, one can stretch different areas of the corpora.

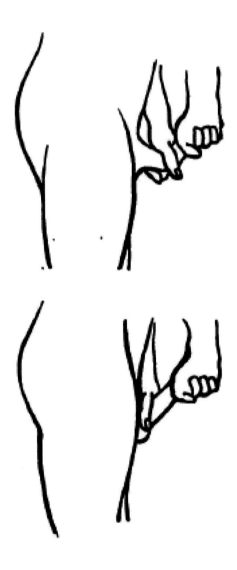

Similarly, one can continue to pull the penis straight out, and cup the bottom of the penis with two to four fingers from the other hand. By lifting straight up, one creates an inverted V. This creates a similarly effective stretch involving the underside of the penis.

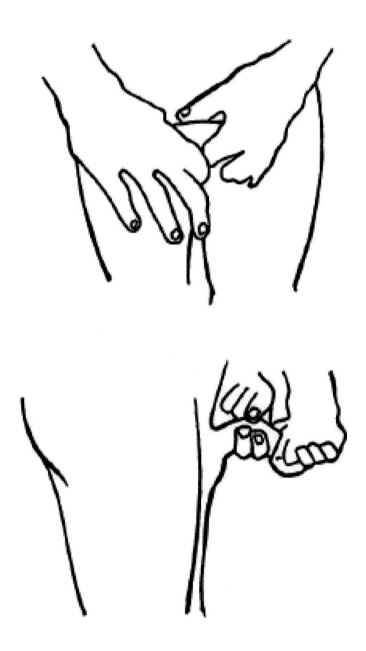

There are many creative forms of stretching that are described on multiple Internet forums. As you can imagine, the penis can be stretched in every imaginable fashion. Furthermore, there are many different schedules and intensities that are recommended. As in bodybuilding, with time, one can increase the intensity and frequency of penis stretching.

One way to increase the intensity is to add a second hand on top of the first hand to generate more power.

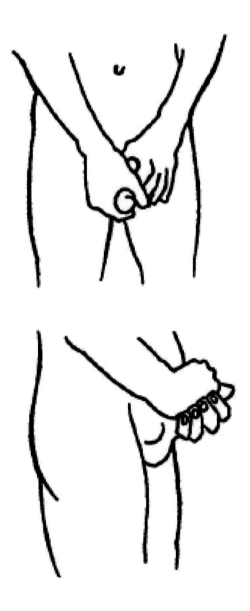

Some advocate for intermittent light quick stretches. For example, one can do very brief and gentle stretches after voiding. If one were to adopt this habit, it would require very little commitment of time or effort. One could also employ this strategy to augment a more formal stretching protocol.

Some of the more elaborate types of exercises employ the use of homemade devices. One creative method involves placement of thick padding over the middle of a drumstick, resting the drumstick over the thighs, and stretching the penis over the device. This would give the penis an inverted-V appearance. In such a fashion, different areas of the ventral (bottom) surface of the penis can be stretched. Obviously, when using this technique, it is important to use a solid drumstick of adequate thickness so as to make sure the drumstick does not break.

Another alternative is to grasp the penis and bend over slightly. Then place the padded drumstick behind the thighs, and bend the dorsal surface of the penis over the padded drumstick. The result of this exercise is to assist in producing a V shape to the penis during the stretch.

A more advanced exercise involves grasping the very proximal penis, behind the scrotum, being very careful to not include the testicles. With the testicles resting in front of the proximal hand, the other hand is placed on the distal shaft. Both hands are pulled upwards, which exerts pressure on the internal penis, as well as the ligaments. It is critical in this stretch that the testicles are not involved, and are in front of the hand. Failure to do so could result in testicular injury.

Does stretching work? There is very little objective data regarding any of these recommendations, and the results are largely anecdotal. No particular schedule is particularly effective or safe. Never perform a stretching exercise with a full erection. Attempting to bend an erect penis can actually result in a fracture type injury which can result in permanent damage.

Advocates of these techniques suggest that mild soreness the following day is common. Most stretches are held from anywhere between 10 seconds and up to five minutes or longer, depending upon comfort.

SECTION 2

General Guidelines For Penis Exercises

Penis exercises including jelking and stretching follow some of the same principles as resistance training. One of these principles is that overtraining is not conducive to maximum gains. In other words, there is not a linear relationship between increasing size and the amount of time spent training. Initially, it is advised that men who perform these types of exercises commit to exercise 15 minutes per day, three days per week. Eventually, this could be increased. Some advocates feel that the gains obtained with these types of exercises may be permanent. Others suggest that after a gain is obtained, the individual should continue to perform light exercises for a period of several months in order to assure that the benefits are maintained.

Bodybuilders gain mass by resting between sessions and gradually increasing the intensity of their exercises. These principles should be followed as well. It is possible to over train. Signs of overtraining include a decrease in sensation or numbness. The development of red spots is a sign of petechia or small hemorrhages. These should resolve spontaneously, but are clearly a sign of doing too much. Proponents of penis exercises state that a mild sense of fatigue after exercising is permissible, decreased sensation is not.

Prior to performing penis exercises, one should warm up the phallus. Heat increases blood flow, which will facilitate the stretching exercises, and make the penis more flexible.

While heat is recommended prior to stretching or jelqing exercises, cold is recommended following a session. This can take the form of a wet cold towel applied after training. Changes in skin color such as red spots or darkening of skin color is an indication that too much pressure or force is being applied. The best strategy to adopt when one sees bruising is to lower the force or frequency of the exercise. If there is a bruise in a particular area, this can be addressed by changing the grip to apply less force to that spot.

There are many superficial veins on the penis end and, hence, it is possible to develop a thrombosis or clot in one of these veins. This is a very different condition then a DVT or deep vein thrombosis which can be associated with a pulmonary embolus or death.

A superficial thrombosis is not a life-threatening condition. These tend to resolve with benign neglect (no intervention). A superficial thrombosis feels like a small cord on the penis. One should be evaluated by a physician if they think that they have developed such a condition and should stop any form of training until it has resolved. It is another sign of over-doing it.

Changes in sensation or numbness are another sure sign of overtraining. Erectile dysfunction or any increased challenges in obtaining an erection should prompt one to back off of any form of penis stretching until the issue has resolved.

SECTION 3

Jelqing

Jelqing is one of the oldest described techniques for penile enlargement. Jelqing likely originated in the Middle East and is a form of milking the penile blood towards the head of the penis for the purpose of enlarging the penis.

Prior to initiating a session of jelqing, it is advised that the penis be warmed for a period of 10 to 15 minutes. This can be done with a warm hot towel, a rice sock as previously described, or with a hot tub. It is advised that this be performed 3 to 5 times a week.

Jelqing is performed with the penis semi-erect, not with a full erection and can be performed in a sitting position or while standing up. One wraps the thumb and forefinger around the penis as if to make the OK sign and gently milks the blood in the penis towards the glans.

This is performed over a period of 2 to 3 seconds and should be performed with the penis lubricated with a product such as KY jelly. This can be performed up to 100 times initially and then progress up to 200 strokes per session.

The goal is to milk the blood from the base of the penis towards the glans penis. The jelq stroke begins next to the pubic bone. Jelqing can be performed in conjunction with hand stretching. It is important to understand that this is absolutely not an exact science. Whatever you do should not hurt. Never do

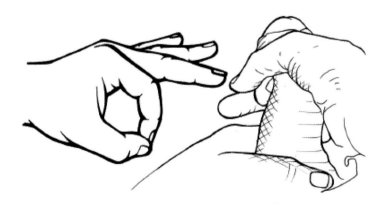

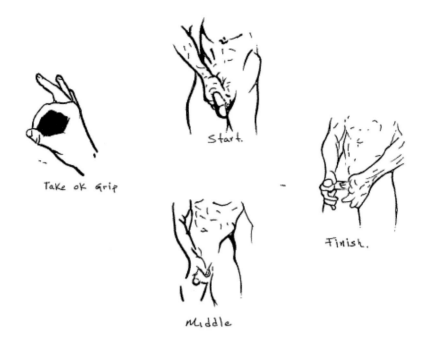

these exercises with a full erection and never perform this if there is any pain. One should not ejaculate while performing this exercise.

Another jelqing technique involves placing the circular OK grip at the base of the penis and then stroking towards the glans penis over a period of 2 to 3 seconds. Prior to completion the second hand restarts this motion at the base of the penis which has the effect of sequentially milking the penis distally.

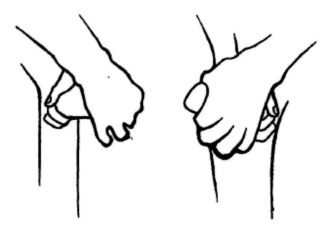

This technique is performed with the penis lubricated and over a 10 to 20 minute period of time. If one develops a full erection during this procedure, then the exercise should be discontinued. It is best to perform this with a partial erection and the frequency can be 2 to 5 days per week. An alternative technique is to start the jelq motion at the head of the penis and stroke back towards the base, which is termed reverse jelqing. Uncircumcised men may benefit from pulling their foreskin back towards the base with one hand before starting the jelq motion.

The goal of jelqing is to fill the corpora cavernosa with blood, and then to increase the pressure within the corpora by forcing the blood up or down the corpora. Theoretically, this may increase the size of the corpora and potentially increase the girth and length.

There have been reports of the development of erectile dysfunction in young patients performing this maneuver. In order to obtain an erection, there is a requirement for both an increase of vascular flow into the penis along with the ability to trap the blood within the corpora cavernosa. Jelqing can potentially injure the mechanism of trapping the blood, which requires passive occlusion of the veins.

The advantage of this technique is that the cost is minimal. The only equipment that is needed is a water-based lubricant. Advocates claim that there may be some results as early as one month.

Most penile exercise regimens suggest that both stretching and jelqing be incorporated. The two techniques are likely complimentary. The stretching may be more beneficial for increasing length, and the jelqing may address girth.

SECTION 4

Edging And Ballooning

Edging is the practice of maintaining an erection for long periods of time without ejaculation in the hopes that this will actually increase the size of the penis. The concept is based upon the belief that extended periods of increased pressure within the corpora cavernosa will increase the volume of the tissue. It is known that patients who become impotent and lose the ability to achieve spontaneous nocturnal erections will experience shrinkage of the penis over a period of time.

There is very little reported literature to support edging, although it's an interesting concept. The term edging is based upon advocates stimulating themselves to the "edge", but not to the point of orgasm. In other words, they receive enough stimulation to come close to achieving a climax but then they stop sexual stimulation to delay the orgasm.

Ballooning is somewhat similar to edging, however, instead of stroking one's penis, one rubs in a circular motion over a discrete spot on the penis. At the same time, it is performed in conjunction with a Kegel exercise. A Kegel exercise is a type of voluntary contraction of the muscles of the pelvis and the anal sphincter. Kegel exercises are commonly performed after women have childbirth, to try to regain urinary control. If a client were to voluntarily interrupt their urinary stream using only the muscles of the pelvis, they would be performing a Kegel exercise. This should be done while continuing to breathe normally.

Ballooning involves continued stimulation of a desirable spot on the penis while performing a Kegel exercise. So the goal of ballooning is to achieve an erection by stimulation of a desirable spot and to force additional blood into the penis with a Kegel contraction. Again, there is little in the way of literature to support this maneuver.

6 Devices

FDA Guidance On Devices

No device currently on the market is approved by the FDA for penile enlargement. In general, medical devices require stringent testing by the food and drug administration. Section 510 of the Federal food drug and cosmetic act allows certain class two devices to be exempt from the usual requirements if they are found to have characteristics of devices within that generic type that are or have been in commercial distribution. Some devices which (illegally) market their ability to enlarge the penis are registered as external penile rigidity devices. According to the FDA, external penile rigidity devices include vacuum pumps, construction rings and penile splints.

External penile rigidity devices are not intended for use for penile enlargement. Therefore, a device may be legally registered with the FDA, but that is not to suggest that the FDA approves of the use of the device for penile enlargement. To suggest that any external device is approved by the FDA for penile enlargement is not only wrong, but also illegal.

Similarly, the FDA does not approve the use of any herbal supplements for erectile dysfunction or penile enlargement. The FDA does regulate the purity and safety of herbal supplements but has limited ability to regulate the veracity of claims made by the manufacturer.

Especially in the area of male enhancement, one needs to be very leery of advertisements seen on the internet. The FDA lacks the manpower to shut down every company with bogus claims. Even when the FDA does act, many companies simply change their address or the names of their products.

SECTION 2

Clamping Of The Penis

The concept of clamping revolves around placing a mechanical ring around the base of the penis which theoretically prevents the outflow of blood from the superficial venous system and at the same time allows arterial blood flow into the penis. The goal of clamping is to increase the girth of the penis; advocates of clamping advise that this be performed with an erection. Sessions can last no longer than 10 minutes, and up to three times per day. In addition, if tingling or numbness occurs, the session should be discontinued immediately. Also, they advise that if the penis becomes black in color that the session be discontinued.

There are no available studies which would indicate efficacy of clamping. There are significant risks associated with this technique. If too much pressure is applied to the delicate nerves, particularly the dorsal nerve, this could result in permanent loss of sensation of the penis. There is also a risk of the development of a thrombus or clot in a vain. Additionally, there is a risk that this technique could also result in irreparable erectile dysfunction.

Excessive pressure placed along the urethra could result in the development of a urethral stricture, a narrowing of the lumen that could impair the flow of the urethra. While most of the self-administered exercises seem relatively safe, clamping may be one of the most dangerous options. If one is insistent upon attempting clamping, be absolutely certain that the device can be easily and quickly removed. Placement of a tight ring around the base of the penis, which can not be removed after the penis is swollen, could result in an absolutely catastrophic result. Most of the available commercial products available for clamping will have a quick release mechanism installed. Other devices utilize a pneumatic (or air pressure) system.

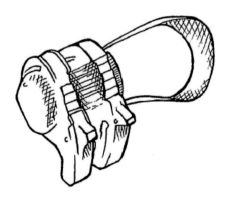

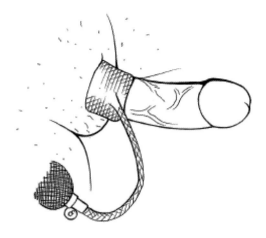

SECTION 3

Vacuum Erection Devices

Vacuum erection devices are commonly used for the treatment of erectile dysfunction. A vacuum-erection device utilizes a cylinder which is placed around the penis, and allows for the creation of a vacuum. The penis becomes engorged as blood is drawn in. The increased penis volume is caused both by arterial inflow as well as venous backflow. Medical grade vacuum-erection devices can cost between $150 and $500.

Some devices utilize a hand held pump to create the vacuum. Other devices utilize a battery- driven mechanical system. The cylinder fits around the base of the penis and, in order to create a proper vacuum, a seal must be created. This can be facilitated by placing KY jelly around the base of the vacuum.

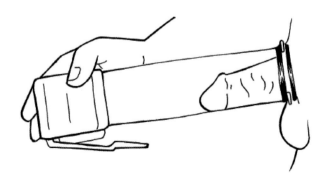

Peer reviewed literature suggests mixed results. Some reports suggest modest gains, while other reports suggest that there were no gains whatsoever.

Vacuum erection devices can be a covered benefit of some insurance carriers when used for the treatment of erectile dysfunction. Prolonged use of a vacuum erection device can increase the pressure in blood vessels and increase the risk of vascular damage. Vacuum erection devices should not be used for more than 30 minutes per session. Too much suction can create permanent injury.

The advantage of vacuum erection devices includes relative safety. Vacuum erection devices have been utilized for the treatment of erectile dysfunction for many years and, assuming that a medical grade device is used within specified time limits, there is relatively little danger. The principal disadvantage of vacuum erection devices is the relative lack of efficacy and failure to demonstrate prolonged gains. It is probably a much better tool for treatment of impotency than it is for penile enlargement.

SECTION 4

Penile Extenders

Penile extenders are mechanical devices which are affixed to two points on the penis externally. The proximal fixation point provides traction against the distal fixation point. The distal point is usually a silicone noose wrapped around the corona, or rim of the glans. The two fixation points are connected by extender rods. By gradually increasing the size of the extender rods, there is progressive increase in traction.

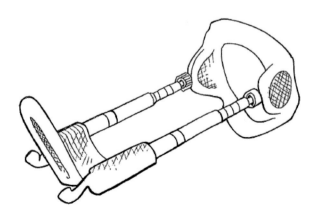

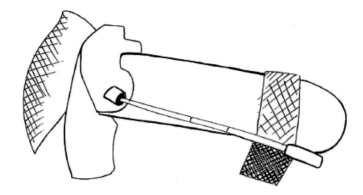

Some devices have small springs inside the extender rods. There is data presented in peer reviewed literature which does, in fact, suggest that there are modest gains associated with these devices. Penile extenders have also been used in the treatment of Peyronie's disease, although they are not FDA approved for this use. However, it is approved as a class one medical device in Europe. Some men have reported gains up to 1.5 inches in length, and some have reported gains in girth as well.

When utilized within parameters, these devices are relatively safe. Costs range between $50 and $400. Some devices are small enough to allow participants to use the device under their clothing in a discreet manner. As such, it may allow patients to actually wear the device at work, facilitating the use of the product for up to 9 hours per day.

As a general rule, it is probably best to use the device initially for a period of 3 hours and then progressively (over a period of 1 to 2 months) the client may increase the time up to 9 hours. This is obviously much less cumbersome than penile weights which must be used with no pants on. On the other hand, less traction may be obtained with an extender than with penile weights. In order to avoid injury to the delicate skin of the penis, be sure to use plenty of padding around the silicone straps employed by extenders. One can place soft padding directly around the penis, as well as around the silicone straps.

Patients who are prone to infection, such as those with uncontrolled diabetes, are prohibited. Those with active infections of the genitalia including sexually transmitted diseases, such as herpes, should not use this product. Also, those with structural abnormalities, such as testicular cancer, hernia or lymphoma should not use a penile extender. Those who have impaired sensation due to stroke, paraplegia or quadriplegia should also not consider use of a penile extender. It should not be used while engaged in sports or while sleeping.

SECTION 5

All Day Stretching (Penile Traction Therapy)

Penis stretching is also referred to as manual stretching. The concept is simple. Stretching the penis all day long may make the organ larger. Creative entrepreneurs have actually developed a number of different devices to facilitate this practice. The penis is stretched in every imaginable fashion- upwards, laterally, and down the leg. Some type of harness is placed around the penis and usually secured under the glans penis proximal to the corona radiata (under the rim of the penis). This harness is attached to a strap which is secured around the client's body. The penis is literally stretched all day long.

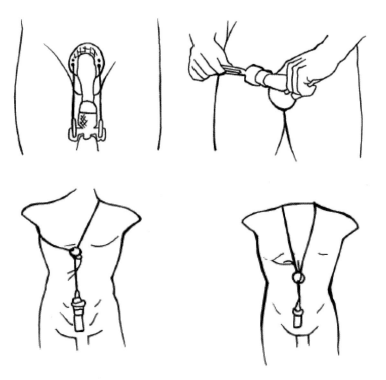

The goal of all-day stretching is to stretch the suspensory ligament, and also the corpus cavernosum and corpus spongiosum. In other words, the goal is to stretch the penis and also to help release the penis from the fixation of the penis to the pubis. The force of the stretch obtained by these devices is similar to penile extenders and the results would be expected to be similar.

Both the all day stretch devices and the penile extenders can be worn discreetly under the clothing. The cost is similar as well, ranging between $100 and $200. There is more literature in peer reviewed journals regarding penile extenders, but the concept of the device is identical. These devices will not exert as much force as can be obtained with penile weights, but may be safer.

SECTION 6

Penis Weight Systems

Some proponents of weight systems advise their clients to exercise up to an hour a day, six days a week. They suggest significant results in six months time or longer. Advocates of this type of system suggest that at least 5 pounds of force must be administered in order to achieve significant benefit. This force is delivered over a 15-minute time frame with subsequent five-minute breaks to allow restoration of normal circulation.

Hindu Sadhus and some African tribes have historically hung rocks from their penis to enlarge it. There is anecdotal evidence that this is highly effective. A theoretical advantage of penis weight systems is an improved ability to apply significant traction to the shaft of the penis. The most delicate part of the penis is the glans. Penile extenders function by applying a noose just proximal to the glans. Attempting to apply more ambitious pressure with a penile extender may result in the creation of blisters at the site that the noose is applied. Penis weight systems are much more aggressive than penis extenders. They certainly are not designed to be worn all day. They are capable of exerting significantly more tension and are designed to be used for 15 minutes at a time with subsequent five-minute breaks.

The amount of weight utilized increases over a period of time. As a general rule, one should start with a weight of 3 pounds and never increase to more then 10 pounds. Penises that are smaller will not be able to accommodate heavier weights. Longer penises can accommodate heavier weights because the pressure or force is dissipated over a greater surface area. Penises less than 4 1/2 inches should not exceed 5 lbs of weight.

Penis weight systems involve wrapping the shaft with material followed by placement of a clamp which is placed circumferentially around the wrapping material. A hook is attached to the clamp and weights are hung from the clamp.

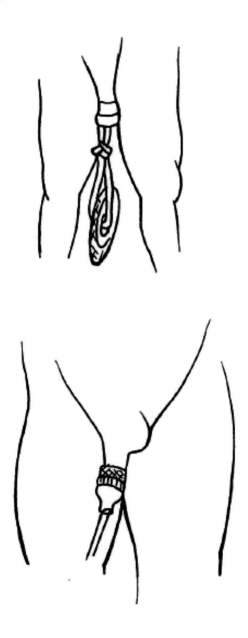

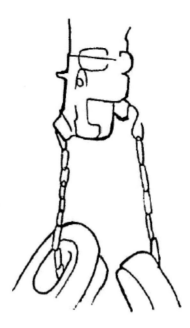

The goal of the system is to distribute the tension across the shaft of the penis, as opposed to using the rim of the penis as a handle. Commercial systems are available at Penis-Weights.com or new optimal.com.

Of the non-surgical treatment options available, penile weights probably have the greatest potential, both for positive gains as well as side effects. This is certainly the most aggressive nonsurgical option. If a client was not careful, there is absolutely a risk of injury. Penile-weight enthusiasts state that the weights should only be used for 15 minutes at a time and there should then be a five minute recovery time.

Some advise clients to use the weights for several hours per day. Most recommend weights of less than 8 pounds, but there are reports of clients using up to 20 pounds after long periods of training. Certainly, if an individual were to notice a change in color, numbness, or a cold penis developing, they should discontinue the exercise. If stretching the tissues of the penis logically could be expected to result in increases in length, and possibly girth, then weights may be more effective than other modalities due to its ability to produce greater traction. Many penis-enlargement surgeons do, in fact, recommend weights following division of the suspensory ligament to prevent subsequent retraction of the penis. If this strategy is effective following surgery, there really is no reason to think that it would not be effective as a sole modality.

The biggest drawback to this form of treatment besides the potential risks is the inconvenience. While penile extenders or all day-stretch devices can potentially be worn discreetly under the clothing at work, weight systems largely require a client to stand with their pants off for long periods of time. This could potentially be a problem for certain occupations. Very few men will be willing to stand virtually naked with 5 pounds of weights hanging from their penis every day for months. Perhaps this is one reason that this practice has not been widely adopted.

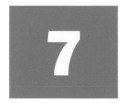

CHAPTER

7 Injection Therapy

Theory behind fillers

The following chapter is devoted to a detailed description of the multiple and varied substances that have been used as fillers of the penis through injection therapy.

All of these fillers are injected into the penis in the area between dartos fascia and Buck's fascia. The purpose of these fillers is to increase the girth of the penis. The fillers may increase the flaccid length of the penis but are unlikely to change the erect length. Fillers are placed in an office setting, under local anesthesia. In order to obtain adequate anesthesia, a short-acting anesthetic agent such is Lidocaine or Marcaine is usually injected into the dorsal nerve of the penis and then a ring block is completed. That means that the anesthetic agent is injected circumferentially around the base of the penis. Local anesthesia is very effective in these types of procedures and is very safe. It obviously is much cheaper to perform these types of procedures under local anesthesia in an office setting, as one does not accrue the cost of an operating room and general anesthesia.

A cannula or small needle is placed beneath the skin with the products placed on the top surface of the penis.

Because no incision is necessary, recovery times tend to be relatively rapid. Dependent upon the specific product, sexual intercourse may be resumed within 4 to 6 weeks or less.

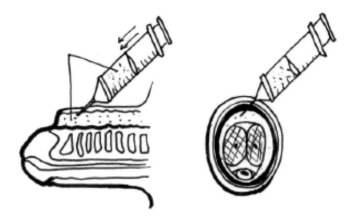

The cost and potential complications are quite variable, dependent upon the product used. Some of the products mentioned are only available in international markets. While some of the products mentioned are FDA approved for medical use, none of the products are specifically indicated for penile enhancement. All of these products are placed into the shaft of the penis. Products placed into the glans penis (glansplasty or glans augmentation) represent a separate category. Some of the products will be very short-acting and are likely to be reabsorbed in as little as six months to a year.

The long-lasting products, particularly PMMA, will not be reabsorbed by the body. While this may seem to be advantageous, there's also an attendant risk, as side effects can be permanent. It can be very difficult, if not impossible, to remove PMMA, and side effects, while rare, can be debilitating. In order to produce a substantial gain in girth, usually at least 20 ml. of material is injected per treatment session. Some of the products may be injected over multiple sessions.

SECTION 2

Collagen

Collagen is the most abundant protein in the human body. It's a substance that holds the whole body together. Collagen is the major large molecule of most connective tissue. It provides strength and structure. 25 to 35% of all of the proteins in the body is collagen. Collagen is created by fibroblasts. Collagen itself can be used as a scaffold for tissue regeneration.

SECTION 3

Injectable Collagen

Some products provide a scaffold, which allows the bodies own fibroblasts to produce natural collagen. An alternative, is to directly inject collagen as a filler (Zyderm and Zyplast are both examples of bovine linked collagen, which is produced in injectable form). Because it is derived from cows, allergy testing is required prior to administration. ,

Very rare cases of localized tissue necrosis can occur in 1 in 10.000 cases due to vascular interruption. Cosmoderm and Cosmoplast are also forms of collagen, but are bioengineered and, as such, do not require a skin test. Collagen is naturally broken down by the body by collagenase. Products that directly inject collagen, like filler, tend to be short- acting. They may have effects that last from a few months to a year; the product usually only lasts 3 to 6 months. Granuloma formation is a possible risk. The risk of a hypersensitivity reaction is less than 1.3%.

SECTION 4

Hyaluronic Acid Including Juvaderm, Restylane, and Perlane

Hyaluronic acid products are among the most popular dermal fillers. Hyaluronic acid is the most common glycosaminoglycan in skin. It binds collagen and elastin fibers. This includes products such as Restylane, Perlane and Juvaderm. Hyaluronic acid is derived from bacteria or rooster combs (the large fleshy skin atop a rooster's head). These products can last up to 12 months. Hyaluronic acid is found in the human body and is a natural component of skin and cartilage. It combines with water to form a gel that swells. It holds cells together in a jell-like matrix.

The product is highly biocompatible, and there have been millions of uses.

Most adverse events associated with hyaluronic acid injections are temporary, and include redness, swelling or localized granulomas. There is a small risk of delayed hypersensitity reactions (1 in 5,000). When utilized to increase the girth of the shaft of the penis, typically 20 ml. or more of the products are injected.

Hyaluronic acid works both by increasing the girth of the phallus, with the volume of material injected, but also has a secondary effect of stimulating subsequent collagen growth. Hyaluronic acid has been known to bring water to the surface of the skin producing a cushion-like effect.

Side effects are relatively few but can include a blue skin discoloration known as the Tyndall effect. If there are untoward side effects secondary to the use of hyaluronic acid, this can be reversed with hyaluronidase. This is like an antidote and represents a unique safety feature.

SECTION 5

Poly-L-Lactic Acid (PLLA)

Sculptra and NewFill are proprietary formulations of (PLLA). NewFill is available in Europe, while Sculptra is FDA approved, and is available in the USA. PLLA is biodegradable, and serves as a scaffold for collagen production. It is composed of micro crystals that recruit fibroblasts to produce natural collagen. It is synthetic and biodegradable. It can be stored for up to 2 years before it is reconstituted.

PLLA is not immunologically active and does not cause allergic reactions. Long term side effects are unlikely, as the product is not permanent. It is broken down with time and replaced by one's own collagen. It is currently used in cosmetic surgery for the treatment of fine lines and wrinkles. It is widely used for off-label uses. One of the complications associated with PLLA is the development of small bumps or granulomas, even years after treatment. Nodules are small bumps, and are common. Sometimes these can be treated with injections of localized steroids.

PLLA is indicated for treatment of AIDS patients that have lipo-atrophy and is useful for producing relatively large-volume defects. The effects of PLLA can take weeks or months to manifest a volume change, but can last for up to two years. This is a relatively safe product that has been utilized in mainstream medicine for many years. Surgeons often use sutures containing PLLA that are naturally absorbed by the body.

SECTION 6

Calcium Hydroxyapatite (Radiesse or ArteFill)

These are FDA approved cosmetic dermal fillers. These products were developed for treatment of skin lines, and are also used in vocal cord surgery and periodontal defects. Calcium hydroxyapatite is a natural substance that is present in the body. The microspheres serve as a framework to stimulate natural collagen growth for up to two years.

This product does not require allergy testing prior to administration. The concept of creating a framework for natural collagen production is similar to that of PMMA (see Chapter 7, Section 8, below), however, this is a temporary product which eventually becomes absorbed by the body. This lasts longer than hyaluronic acid derivatives, but it is not permanent. The effects are immediate as the gel increases the girth of the penis, and persists as collagen is produced between the microspheres.

There is very little risk of an allergic reaction, as this is a substance that is naturally found within the body. There is a risk of migration of the product, which is tempered by the fact that the effects of the product are temporary. The product is likely to be metabolized over 10 to 14 months, although some patients may absorb it much quicker, in 6 to 9 months.

SECTION 7

Cymetra and Megafill

Cymetra is micronized AlloDerm, which can be injected. Cymetra is an FDA approved product available in the USA. Megafill is micronized acellular dermis available only in Korea at this time. They are highly processed, commercially available products obtained from a tissue bank. It serves as a scaffold, which is replaced by the patient's own tissue. In other words, the products is a type of biologic scaffold and depends upon tissue engineering to ultimately be replaced by the patients own tissues. When implanted into a patient, both tissue growth and revascularization have been observed.

The patient's own fibroblasts produce collagen and promote regeneration of tissue with the structure being provided by the injected material. It is critical that patients who receive this product perform appropriate postoperative physiotherapy to keep the fluid material in the intended position; meaning, it is possible for the material to migrate in an uneven distribution unless proper care is taken. When compared in durability to Zyplast, Cymetra has been shown to be superior, with longer-lasting benefit.

SECTION 8

PMMA

PMMA has a very long track record as a dermal filler. Polymethylmethacrylate is a plastic- processed polymer that is composed of microspheres. The concept behind the use of PMMA is to stimulate natural collagen formation by stimulating one's own fibroblasts.

The PMMA is not absorbed. It has been approved by the FDA as permanent facial filler. It has been used as cement in ENT surgery, neurosurgery, and joint replacement surgery. It can only be removed by cutting it out. The PMMA is combined with a filling agent, which provides for immediate increase in volume. Over time, the associated filler degrades and, that volume deficit is compensated for by production of one's own collagen around the PMMA.

This product does have accepted use in mainstream medicine. For instance, it is used in spine surgery and also for treatment of GERD. However, its use in penile enlargement is very controversial. PMMA is usually combined with some other substance and is not delivered in its purest form.

Artefill is an FDA approved substance which contains 20% PMMA and 3.5%collagen. The collagen is from an animal source (bovine) and, as such, it is necessary to perform a skin test prior to the use of Artefill to make sure that the patient is not allergic.

All products that utilize bovine-linked collagen require a skin test prior to administration. This is generally performed two weeks prior to use of the product. Artefill is commercially available in the United States, and is approved as a medical device for the correction of smile lines. In 1 ml. of ArteFill, there are roughly 6,000.000 particles of PMMA. Because it is bovine-linked, there is a risk of allergy, and patients who undergo such an injection require double-skin testing prior. A similar product is Artecoll which is also PMMA and collagen and is available in Mexico. This was first introduced in Europe, and has a granuloma rate of less than .1%.

There are a variety of other products containing PMMA with other carriers that are available abroad. Metacrill is available in Mexico and Brazil and contains PMMA and Carboxymethylcellulose. It does not require pretesting (no bovine-linked collagen). Linnea Safe contains Hydroxyethylcellulose and PMMA. It is available in Brazil.

Lipen10 is PMMA cross-linked with Dextran. This product is only available in Korea. Artesense is PMMA-linked with collagen available in Brazil. When PMMA is utilized in penile enlargement, generally 20 ml.

or more are utilized. This usually requires 4 to 6 punctures with a needle or a cannula.

PMMA is a type of synthetic injectable filler. PMMA acts as a foreign body in the tissues and, as such, elicits a host response to try to remove the gel. Inflammatory granulomas may develop at the site of injection. This reaction can occur many years later. In addition to inflammatory nodules, the development of fibrosis or scarring is a risk. The inflammatory nodules can occur up to six years after injection. Together these phenomena can result in tissue contracture and tissue hardening. In addition, a thick capsule can form around the PMMA which is quite resistant to treatment.

One can develop necrosis of the skin. Some patients develop chronic inflammation which may be permanent. Along with these problems, some patients have chronic bleeding or chronic pain. Uneven distribution of the product can result in an uneven or lumpy penis. There can be necrosis or death of the overlying skin as well. While PMMA offers the advantage of being relatively minimally invasive and potentially durable, the profound risks of chronic-delayed problems have discouraged all but a few practitioners from attempting this form of therapy.

SECTION 9

Silicone

Small doses of medical-grade silicone have historically been successfully utilized in cosmetic surgery in very small doses. The doses that have been used have been less than 1 ml. In order to achieve successful penile augmentation, much larger doses are required.

The risks associated with silicone injection in the penis include the risk of migration of the product, swelling, and granulomatous reaction. Migration of silicone has reported to cause pneumonitis or inflammation of the lungs. There is also a risk of damaging blood vessels and nerves in the penis resulting in erectile dysfunction or much worse.

There have been multiple-reported cases of death secondary to injection of silicone by unqualified practitioners. Some of these practitioners have injected industrial grade silicone as opposed to medical-grade silicone which is unconscionable. Medical-grade silicone for injection is only available to surgeons for experimental purposes.

While some of the fillers used in penile augmentation are controversial, there is no controversy about the use of silicone. There is absolute agreement that the use of silicone for penile augmentation is absolutely contraindicated. Nobody should ever consider silicone injection for their penis.

SECTION 10

Glansplasty

Glansplasty involves the injection of a hyaluronic acid derivative into the glans penis. Some refer to this as getting your helmet pumped up. The material is injected between the epithelial layer and the corpus spongiosum. A total of 2-3ml. of material is injected through multiple individual puncture sites. The puncture sites allow for distribution of hyaluronic acid by injecting the material in a fan like pattern through each puncture.

The material is actually injected into the lamina propria mucosa. The patient satisfaction rate was 77% in one study.

In addition to increasing the circumference of the glans penis, there may be a secondary benefit. This procedure may reduce sensitivity of the glans, which can provide benefit for patients suffering from premature ejaculation. This effect is powerful enough that some physicians perform this procedure purely for the purposes of delaying ejaculation.

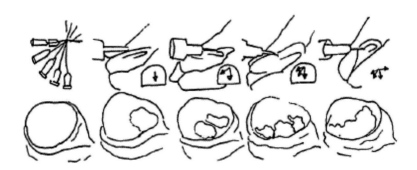

8 Surgery

Incision Of The Suspensory Ligament (Ligamentolysis)

Approximately 50% of the total length of the penis resides within the body. Part of the penis is attached to the pubis by the suspensory ligament. The suspensory ligament has a superficial branch, which is referred to as the fusiform or falciform ligament. The deeper branch of the suspensory ligament is referred to as the arcuate or triangular ligament.

The neurovascular bundle of the penis, which includes the dorsal nerve of the penis, sits on top of the penis in the midline. For this reason, it is best to cut the suspensory ligament immediately adjacent to the pubis, as opposed to cutting the ligament next to the penis. Cutting the ligament too close to the penis could result in loss of sensation of the penis. The ligaments can either be cut with scissors or with a laser. Cutting the ligament allow a penis to be pulled outward. The change in length following such surgery is 1-3 cm. (about 1 inch). The risk of cutting the ligament is that the penis loses some structural support. This changes the angle of the penis when it is erect.

In addition, the penis becomes more low-lying. Another potential risk is that the penis can subsequently reattach to the undersurface of the pubis. Paradoxically, this can actually potentially result in shortening of the penis. Various strategies have been employed to try to reduce the risk of reattachment of the penis to the pubis. Some surgeons try to place some of the patient's own fat under the pubis to prevent reattachment. The fat can be harvested from the adjacent spermatic cord. Some surgeons have attempted to place a prosthetic device under the pubis to prevent reattachment.

Almost every surgeon recommends that some form of physiotherapy be performed in the postoperative period. This can take the form of traction devices, or penile weights in order to try to prevent reattachment of the penis to the pubis.Incision of the suspensory ligament is usually performed through a small incision just above the penis. This can either be an inverted V incision or a transverse incision. Incision of the suspensory ligament is commonly performed in conjunction with girth procedures.

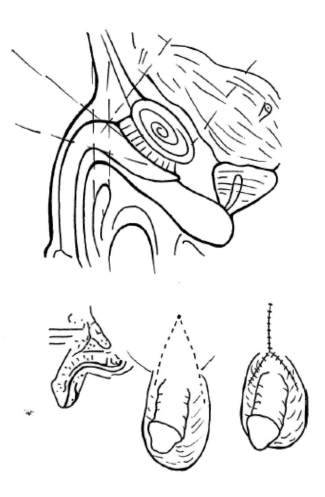

Most commonly, this is done at the same time as the incision of the ligament, although some surgeons prefer to perform these as two separate procedures. Patient satisfaction rates tend to be low, approaching 30 to 35%, and even lower in patients with penile dysmorphic disorder. Potential complications include sexual dysfunction. The cost of this procedure is between $4,000 and $7,000.

SECTION 2

Inverted VY Plasty

After cutting the suspensory ligament, the penis hangs in a lower position. The purpose of the inverted VY plasty is to prevent the skin from tethering the penis and preventing it from hanging in its more dependent position. Ideally, the inverted VY plasty allows for the relocation of the skin and produces additional vertical length. An alternative to the inverted VY plasty is to make a transverse incision and then close this incision again in such a way as to create additional length.

Performing such a maneuver can create complications. This can result in the advancement of suprapubic hairy skin onto the shaft of the penis. Specifically, there may be a scar referred to as a keloid. Some patients may be more prone towards keloid formation, particularly those who have had difficulty with wound healing in the past. In addition to keloid formation, the VY flaps can fail if not created in a technically efficient manner, such as if the flaps are too thick.

Another risk is that of scrotalization, in which a low-lying penis seems to emanate from the scrotum. Some surgeons prefer to make a simple

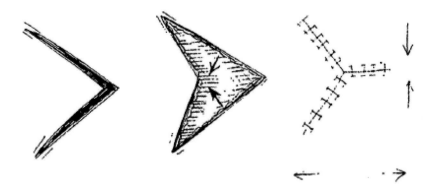

transverse incision and to depend upon subsequent physiotherapy such as skin stretching to allow for proper wound healing. In other words, they make a 1-inch sideways incision just above the penis rather than the more elaborate inverted V incision. The simple sideways incision is less likely to have difficulty healing, but requires additional post-operative care in order to allow the penis to hang outside of the body.

SECTION 3

Free Fat Transfer

Historically, free fat transfer has been one of the mainstays of surgical enhancement of the penis. Free fat transfer involves removal of fat from either the pre-pubic area or the inner thighs with subsequent transfer of this fat to the penis. When fat is removed from the area around the penis, this alone can be beneficial from a cosmetic standpoint as this may give the penis the appearance of being longer.

The transfer of free fat has gained wide-spread acceptance among plastic surgeons and is commonly used in facelift surgery. Fat grafting has proven to be a safe and effective procedure for enhancing tissue defects. Recently, free fat transfer has been popularized for breast augmentation, and seems to be gaining in popularity.

The results obtained with free fat transfer are operator dependent. The results vary widely, dependent upon the skill of the surgeon, the equipment used for harvesting, the equipment used for cleansing and processing of the lipoaspirate and the technique used for reinjection. There are obviously many different variables, and, if meticulous attention is not paid to every single aspect, a poor result will be the outcome.

In the early days of penile enlargement surgery, a number of surgeons harvested fat and injected this into the penis in a sloppy haphazard fashion. This resulted in irregular absorption of the fat, which led to irregularly shaped, grotesque penises. This led to penis enlargement surgery developing a terrible reputation within mainstream medicine. Free fat transfer is currently widely accepted among plastic surgeons. The results are uniform and predictable using modern techniques.

The initial step in free fat transfer involves preparation of the area from which the fat will be obtained, usually the pre-pubic area above the penis. Tumescence is obtained by infiltrating the area with dilute anesthetic, and tunnels are created with a blunt cannula. A suction apparatus is connected to a small cannula, and an aspirate is obtained.

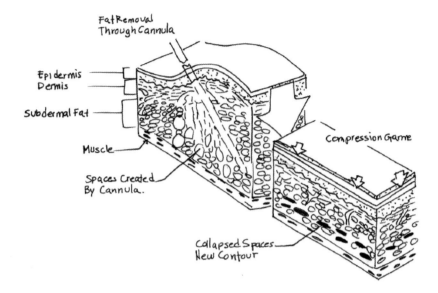

Fat Removal
Through Cannula

Epidermis
Dermis

Subdermal Fat

Muscle

Spaces Created
By Cannula.

Compression Garme

Collapsed Spaces
New Contour

The goal is for the subsequent fat to be transferred and survive. The manner in which the aspirate is processed is critical to this survival. Injecting nonviable fat is unacceptable, as that would result in an irregular, lumpy penis.

There is an underlying principle in plastic surgery which is to "replace like with like". Certainly using one's own fat to increase the girth of the penis is an attractive alternative. The limiting factor is survival of the fat. Modern technology and advancements of surgical techniques has allowed for increased survival of the transferred fat and subsequent improvement in results.

While some of the early pioneers in penile enhancement surgery experienced significant complications from free fat transfer, those results do not necessarily reflect upon modern results with appropriately trained surgeons. However, possible complications still include scarring, nodularity and lumps. There is still a risk that some or all of the fat will not survive.

SECTION 4

Dermal Fat Graft

The most superficial layer of the skin is the epidermis. The deeper layer includes the dermis and subcutaneous' tissues, including fat. When using dermal fat grafts for penile augmentation, the deeper aspect of skin is transferred and used to augment the shaft of the penis. The dermal fat is usually harvested from the crease under the buttocks. This requires at least one or two additional incisions, which obviously adds additional pain and risks of additional potential wound healing problems. This will add additional time to any surgery, and, as such, increases operating room costs. Advantages include increased survival rates compared to free fat transfer.

Some surgeons feel that the increased risks of the additional incisions are too high and use allografts such as Belladerm or Alloderm as alternatives. These products are expensive and add $4,000 to $5,000 to the cost of the procedure. These products are derived from donated human tissue and are distributed through tissue banks.

SECTION 5

Acellular Homologous Grafts Including Belladerm And Alloderm, Acellular Xenografts

Alloderm and Belladerm are derived from donated human skin. They are highly processed, commercially available products obtained from a tissue bank. These are FDA approved products that are used for a variety of medical purposes. They can be used for wound healing. Because they are meticulously processed, there has never been a reported case of transmitted infection from these products.

Alloderm and Belladerm are placed in the space between dartos fascia and Buck's fascia, similar to other thickening products. These come as sheets of tissue and, as such, require placement through one or two surgical incisions.

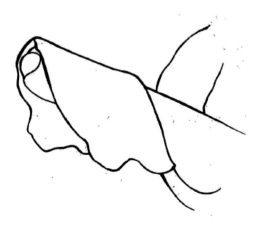

Some surgeons place an incision at the base of the penis, while other surgeons add a second incision just proximal to the glans penis. These products are typically placed on the dorsal (or top) surface of the penis and not ventrally around the corpus spongiosum.

As penile enlargement surgery has evolved, allografts have taken the place of dermal fat graphs for some surgeons. The advantage of an allograft is that it does not require the harvesting of material from other areas of the body, and therefore, reduces the amount of surgery and the amount of incisions. On the other hand, allografts are very expensive, adding thousands of dollars to the cost of girth enhancement.

An allograft is a type of surgical implant. Since the allograft is acellular, it serves as a scaffold or matrix, which is eventually replaced by the patient's own tissue. An allograft can only be placed one time.

The placement of an allograft in the penis is associated with some risks. The penile skin is very thin and covers over the allograft. The greatest risk is that this is can become necrotic and die. This is catastrophic. When this occurs, the allograft must be removed and it may be necessary to place a skin graft on top of the defect. Other risks include the risk of allograft failure or the risk of infection.

There may be a small risk of the development of erectile dysfunction following placement of such a graft. The superficial and deep dorsal nerve lies under the graft. A small risk is that the allograft can contract as it heals which could result in shortening of the penis.

There are also reports of favorable results utilizing a porcine (derived from a pig), acellular graft (which is termed a xenograft). Xenografts (derived from different species) have also been successfully used in other arenas in medicine, such as in the treatment of burn victims.

SECTION 6

Penile Implants

Penile implants are medical devices that are placed into the corpora cavernosa for the purposes of restoring erectile function. Penile implants are either malleable or inflatable. While penile prosthetics are highly effective in restoring man's ability to engage in sexual intercourse, they absolutely do not increase penile size; in fact, quite to the contrary. Many men who undergo implantation surgery are disappointed that there is a reduction in the size of their phallus following surgery. One study found that 72% of men who undergo implantation experience a reduction in stretched penile length.

Counseling patients to expect some reduction in size is included in most urologist's preoperative counseling with implantation patients. In addition to anticipating some reduction in size with implantation of penile implants, removal of such a device is often met with more extreme loss in length. The erectile tissue of the corpora cavernosa becomes fibrotic after the implant is removed, and the loss in length can be dramatic.

Knowing that some loss in length following implantation is common, some urologists have adopted a strategy of trying to maximize preoperative length. As urologists are very familiar with vacuum erection devices, these are commonly recommended, although other devices (including penile extenders) may be more effective.

There is a special category of penile implants which are placed outside of the corpora cavernosa intended to increase the girth of the penis. This implant (the Elist implant) is placed in the same area as fillers, between dartos fascia and Buck's fascia . The device is registered with the FDA and has received 510(K) clearance.

510 (K) clearance implies that the device is substantially equivalent to devices previously classified. This device was cleared to correct soft tissue deformities and aid in the reconstructive process.

There is a fundamental difference between the Elist implant and penile prosthetics utilized for erectile dysfunction. Penile prosthetics are placed into the corpora cavernosa. They are covered over by the thick capsule of the tunica albuginea. The Elist implant is placed outside of this area, closer to the skin, potentially making it somewhat vulnerable to erosion. At this time, Dr. Elist is the only surgeon implanting the device. The total cost for the implant and surgery is $12,000.

SECTION 7

Ventral Phalloplasty

Some men are born with a web attaching their penis to the scrotum. This is a congenital condition. A scrotal web is identified by lifting the penis straight up and observing if it is tethered to the scrotum. Correction of this web is a relatively simple surgical procedure which is illustrated.

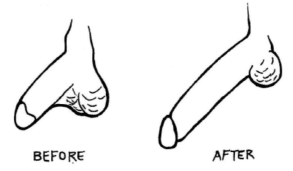

BEFORE   AFTER

A ventral phalloplasty is performed with an asymmetric V incision. This can be performed as an isolated procedure or in conjunction with other surgical procedures including placement of a penile prosthesis. The procedure does not result in an actual increase in erect penile length, but presents the appearance of a longer phallus, which is more separated from the scrotum.

SECTION 8

Saphenous Vein Graft

Harvesting of the saphenous vein in the leg is a rather elaborate operation designed to increase the girth of the penis. The corpora cavernosa are the two cylinders that fill with blood to create on erection. The corpora cavernosa are filled with soft tissue and surrounded by a thick capsule called the tunica albuginea.

Incisions are made in the tunica albuginea of the corpora cavernosa, and the defects that are created are filled with the harvested vein from the leg. This procedure is designed to increase the girth of the penis. This increase occurs only during erections and has been shown to increase the girth of the penis by approximately 1.5 cm. in the erect phallus. This is a very delicate operation, which requires precision to avoid nerve injury which could result in erectile dysfunction. This operation has not gained widespread popularity, although patient satisfaction rates have been high.

SECTION 9

PRP, Regenerative Medicine

Regenerative medicine is a new branch of medicine that deals with tissue engineering and molecular biology. The purpose is to replace or regenerate human cells, tissues and organs or establish normal function.

The use of platelet-rich plasma has achieved widespread popularity within multiple arenas of medicine. Platelet-rich plasma is based upon removing one's own blood, centrifuging the contents, and utilizing the component, which is rich in platelets.

The machines utilized to obtain PRP are FDA approved, as are the kits that the machines utilize. PRP is very safe, as it relies upon the patient's own blood. As such, there is no risk of an allergic reaction. PRP has achieved its greatest popularity in the areas of athletic injuries and pain management. Proponents of PRP cite the benefits of a natural process which uses the body to heal the body. PRP contains multiple growth factors which are the theoretical basis for use in tissue repair. Among the growth factors are PDGF, PDAF, TGF, FGF, ILGF 1&2, Endothelial Growth Factor and Keratinocyte Growth Factor. PRP needs to be activated with either calcium chloride or thrombin.

Theoretically, PRP may stimulate stem cells. Stem cells have the ability to develop into many different types of cells. There have literally been thousands of papers written on the use of PRP with no serious side effects identified to date.

Regenerative medicine is clearly in its very early stages and all of the science and clinical possibilities are not known at this time. PRP is utilized by many hair transplant surgeons in hopes of stimulating stem cells and promoting hair growth. Hair transplant surgeons commonly use PRP at the time of transplantation of hair follicles. They also use it to aid in the healing of the incision line.

As in many other areas of medicine, there are not compelling controlled prospective studies at this time. Many famous athletes such is Kobe Bryant, Alex Rodriguez, Zack Greinke and Peyton Manning have all utilized PRP during their recovery from injuries. One very famous orthopedic surgeon recently stated "I don't know how it works, but I know it works."

There is very little data to suggest that PRP used as a sole modality will increase penile size. There may be some rationale to rejuvenating the tissues of the corpora cavernosa with PRP to enhance erectile function. On a theoretical basis, there may be an increase in mesenchymal stem cells in processed lipoaspirate obtained in free fat transfer. Some surgeons combine PRP with the stem-cell rich lipoaspirate to try to promote new tissue growth. However, at this time, it not clear if the addition of growth factors results in improved survival of the transferred fat. This seems very promising, but again, has not been well studied at this time.

SECTION 10

Polylactic Glycolic Acid. PLGA Scaffold

Polylactic glycolic acid (PLGA) can be used as a scaffold to provide structural support for tissue engineering. PLGA is biodegradable. These are microspheres that are fused together to form a scaffold. This supports cell attachment and proliferation in a controlled manner. This is FDA approved for certain applications, although penis enlargement is not one of them. PLGA can act as a scaffold for transplanted stem cells or cultured cells.

Presently, PLGA can be implanted as a sheet surgically or injected as microparticles. The concept is to obtain cells from the patient and expand these cells in culture. The PLGA scaffold is implanted along with the cultured cells. Eventually, the scaffolds are absorbed over a period of four months. These scaffolds (which are somewhat rigid) are replaced by growth of the cultured cells. This form of tissue engineering is currently available in Belgrade, and Serbia. This does require brief hospitalization and the cost is between $8,000 and $12,000.

The theory of tissue engineering is very elegant and attractive. At the present time, however, the long-term gains have not been all that favorable. Tissue engineering is likely to assume a bigger role in penis enlargement in the future, but at the present time the role is limited.

SECTION 11

Postoperative Instructions

Postoperative instructions will vary dependent upon the details of the procedure. You should always listen to the instructions of your surgeon. Also, you should receive both oral and written instructions and refer to these frequently. In addition, never hesitate to contact your doctor if things don't seem right. Examples would include excessive swelling, problems with an incision, or excessive pain. Fever should always be evaluated.

In general, one should not plan on resuming vigorous physical activity for one month. Sexual activity should not resume until pain has resolved, which may be up to 6 weeks. It is critical to perform post operative stretching after incision of the suspensory ligament. If this is not performed, it is likely that the penis will reattach to the pubis. Paradoxically, this can result in a shorter penis than prior to the operation.

It is also important to massage the penis post operatively for those undergoing procedures to increase girth. Failure to do so can result in a lumpy penis with uneven distribution of the product injected. Massage should be performed with lubrication.

Most patients who undergo ligamentolysis, or division of the suspensory ligament will be asked to perform physiotherapy following surgery. This may involve use of penile weights or a penile extender. This is usually started after the incision has adequately healed. Failure to perform this could result in subsequent shortening of the penis. Always check with your surgeon regarding timing of the initiation of such treatment.

CHAPTER

9 Going Forward With Caution

SECTION 1

Finding A Provider

There are very few American physicians who are willing to perform penile enhancement surgery given their potential exposure to litigation. Subsequently, many who are willing to venture into this arena will choose relatively safe but unproven and less effective options (PRP).

The largest published series of penile enlargement surgeries come from outside the US. In addition, some of the products utilized for penile injection therapy are not available, or are much more expensive in the US. That is not to say that excellent effective treatment is unavailable in the United States. However, male enhancement is much more common internationally and tends to be significantly less expensive. Penile lengthening in conjunction with girth enhancement may cost $15,000 to $20,000 in the USA, compared to well less than half abroad.

Having surgery performed abroad carries certain significant risks. Depending upon the country selected, the hospitals may not have the same standards as American hospitals. Some countries have standards that are identical to those of the United States and medical tourism is a driving force in the local economy. In fact, some American insurance carriers encourage their patients to have certain types of procedures overseas. On the other hand, if a complication should arise from a penile enlargement procedure performed abroad, a patient may have great difficulty finding a local provider willing to care for them. Traveling back to a provider in an exotic location may be time consuming and expensive. In the unfortunate event that a provider is negligent, it may be very difficult to obtain subsequent compensation.

77

In general, penile enlargement should only be performed by a certified urologist or plastic surgeon. If a complication should arise, you want a doctor who is capable of fixing whatever the problem is. Any procedure can have a complication, the majority of which can be managed. You must have a physician who is both available, and capable of addressing any problems that can arise from a procedure.

Questions and actions:

1) What procedure do you plan on performing?
2) What results can I reasonably expect to obtain?
3) Where will the procedure be performed?
4) What are common complications?
5) What are some of the rare complications?
6) How many of these procedures have you personally performed?
7) Where did you learn to perform this procedure?
8) What will be my post operative requirements?
9) When can I return to work?
10) When can I resume sexual intercourse?
11) Should I use a traction device or penile weights after the operation?
12) Who do I call if there is a problem after the procedure? Are you going to give me your cell phone number?
13) What will be my personal cost if there is a requirement for a revision procedure?
14) Am I a good candidate for this procedure?
15) Can I talk to one or more of your patients who has had this procedure previously?
16) Is financing available?
17) Do I need to put a down payment before surgery? What happens if I change my mind?

SECTION 2

Lack Of Mainstream Acceptance

Your local family doctor, urologist, plastic surgeon likely will not endorse any form of penile enlargement. The traditional teaching among specialty organizations and organized medicine in general is that penile enlargement is unnecessary and not effective. Both the American Society of Plastic Surgeons and the American Urology Association do not sanction this form of surgery, except for true micropenis (.6% of all men).

Penile enhancement surgery is not taught as part of any traditional residency program. It is not featured in any standard textbook in urology or plastic surgery. Very few physicians have any type of formal exposure to this surgery.

It is widely recognized that penile dysmorphia is quite prevalent. Although recent technical advances have markedly improved outcomes, the pioneers in this field faced huge obstacles and the outcomes were terrible. Compared to other forms of plastic surgery, patient satisfaction rates tend to lag behind. In some surgeries, the overall patient satisfaction rate was as low as 35%. Performing an operation which is not sanctioned by major professional organizations puts the operating physician in a position where he is very vulnerable to litigation. Particularly in America, most physicians do not wish to assume such risks.

Even though many respected physicians do not advocate this form of elective treatment does not necessarily mean it's not right for you. Some patients do benefit from treatment. Some patients who receive treatment do receive significant physical changes which are permanent. This physical change may engender changes in body image and self-confidence. It is critical that patients be allowed to make informed decisions regarding this highly personal issue. It is certainly not helpful to automatically dismiss these concerns. Because of many physicians lack of knowledge and personal discomfort with the subject matter, many patients turn to the internet for answers. This is evidenced by countless blogs and unscrupulous websites.

Providers must be absolutely vigilant in assuring that patients have realistic goals in their treatment. Patients should know what expected gains can be anticipated. They should also know what the satisfaction rates are based on prior patient outcomes. They must know about anticipated costs as well as likely complications. If something seems too be good to be true, it is.

SECTION 3

Beware Of Charlatans

The desire to lengthen and thicken the penis has inspired many creative and many dangerous options. The Topinama of Brazil has been known to sustain snakebites to the penis to allow the affected organ to be swollen for up to six months. If some guys are willing to undergo a snakebite to the penis, one can only imagine just how far others are willing to go to achieve this goal.

Because there is so little published medical literature in this field, various marketers and charlatans have been presented a tremendous opportunity to exploit men desperate to enlarge their penis.

Probably the most famous case of the nefarious practices of penile enlargement charlatans involved the product Enzyte. This was originally manufactured by Berkeley Premium Natraceuticals of Cincinnati, Ohio. This product claimed it produced natural male enhancement by increasing blood flow. I'm sure you remember "Smilin' Bob" who was always smiling because of his presumably enormous penis. At one time, Enzyte was so popular that they actually had a car entered in NASCAR events. However, the company came under close scrutiny from various governmental agencies due largely to the product's lack of effectiveness. Ultimately, the company's CEO, Steve Warshak, was served with a 112-count criminal indictment and sentenced to prison. The company conceded that it had no scientific studies to support its claims when its feet were held to the fire.

Keep in mind that products that are labeled herbal products do not require the same type of testing by the FDA as prescription medication that require extensive proof of effectiveness before approval. To think that any pill, acting alone, could make a select body part grow is absurd. The fact that Steve Warshak was able to accumulate over $500 million in assets selling this product speaks to the enormous market interested in penile enlargement. It is simply not logical to think that any pill can selectively make a body part grow as an isolated strategy.

In 1994, Congress passed the Dietary Supplement Health and Education Act. This Act enables companies that manufacture herbal supplements to make claims regarding products without proof of efficacy, which of course is quite different from prescription medication. There are now more than 30,000 herbal supplement products. Among the most popular of these products are penile enlargement pills. It is estimated that Americans spend nearly one billion dollars a year on penile enhancement pills. Just as a no magical pill will give an individual a bodybuilder's physique alone, there is no pill that will transform your penis by itself.

SECTION 4

Surgery Gone Bad

Dr. Melvin Rosenstein performed 5,000 to 7,000 penoplasty procedures during a period of time in the 1990s. He was self-proclaimed Dr. Dick.

He performed many of the procedures before the technology was fully developed. His volume of cases was enormous, 5 to 10 cases per day. Eventually, he faced a mountain of lawsuits and retired from penile enlargement surgery.

A famous case involved Dr. Ricardo Samitier who had the misfortune of performing a penoplasty on a man on anticoagulant therapy who bled excessively, had cardiac arrest and died. Dr. Samitier was convicted of manslaughter. A doctor performed an operation that went bad and actually was convicted of manslaughter!

In addition to certified surgeons having misadventures, there are periodic reports of nonmedical doctors taking it upon themselves to inject industrial-grade silicon into the penis. These cases resulted in highly publicized criminal convictions that cast an unfortunate shadow over the entire field of penile enlargement. In addition, some men have been known to self-inject Vaseline or other types of oil-based products into the penis themselves to increase girth. This has resulted in severely deformed penises and other terrible complications.

SECTION 5

Last Minute Tricks

There are a couple of very simple tricks a man can employ to make himself instantly look larger. Just as bodybuilders will do some resistance training immediately before appearing on stage, some physical stimulation of the penis applied immediately before making "an appearance" may paint one in a more favorable light. This trick is certainly employed by a number of penis enlargement surgeons when presenting pictures of select patients before and after surgery. Often the preoperative pictures are flaccid and the postoperative pictures are partially erect.

Another simple trick is that of manscaping. Trimming the pubic hair will not only be more cosmetically appealing, but will actually give the illusion of increased size. When there isn't any underbrush the tree looks taller.

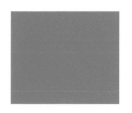

Appendage

COMPARATIVE ANALYSIS OF PENILE ENLARGEMENT OPTIONS

1: Treatment: Over the counter herbal supplements.
Description: Nonprescription natural product.
Potential benefits: It may augment other treatments and facilitate growth, may improve sexual desire or facilitate erections.
Risks: Rare interactions with prescription drugs, some side effects are dose-dependent, many claims are unproven in human trials.
Costs: $20-100/month

2: Treatment: Testosterone
Description: Prescribed medication which can be delivered with intramuscular injections, pellets, patches or cream.
Potential benefits: May increase libido, may have a role in treatment of erectile dysfunction, increase in energy, muscle mass, may facilitate benefits of stretching.
Risks: Shown to not increase penile size after puberty; increased cardiac risk; risk of deep venous thrombosis, promotion of prostate cancer.
Costs: $50-500/month

3: Treatment: Penile stretching exercises.
Description: Exercises performed 3 to 5 times per week; involves hand-stretching the penis in various directions with variable degrees of tension.
Potential benefits: May loosen the ligaments and allow part of the internal penis to externalize; may lengthen the penis as well.

Risks: Minor bruising; clotting of superficial veins; temporary erectile dysfunction; temporary soreness. Lack of studies in peer reviewed literature.
Cost: Minimal

4: **Treatment:** Jelqing.
Description: Using the thumb and index finger to make an "OK" sign, and milking the blood in the penis from the base to the tip.
Potential benefits: May increase length and girth.
Risks: Minor bruising, soreness, erectile dysfunction. Lack of studies in peer reviewed literature.
Cost: Minimal

5: **Treatment:** Edging.
Description: Persistent stimulation of the penis without reaching orgasm.
Potential benefit: May augment other treatments to increase length and girth, may assist in management of premature ejaculation.
Risks: Risk of priapism in patients prone to this condition such as sickle cell carriers.
Cost: Minimal

6: **Treatment:** Ballooning.
Description: Persistent stimulation of a desired spot on the penis, in conjunction with Kegle exercise.
Potential Benefit: May augment other treatments to increase length or girth.
Risks: Lack of studies in peer reviewed literature
Cost: Minimal

7: **Treatment:** Vacuum erection devices.
Description: A cylinder is connected to either a hand held or mechanical pump. The penis is expanded as blood is drawn into the vasculature.
Potential benefits: Gains in length; potential aid in treatment of erectile dysfunction. This may be a covered benefit by many carriers when prescribed for treatment of erectile dysfunction.

Risks: Mild soreness, bruising. Studies indicate negligible to minimal increases in length
Cost: $100-500

8:     **Treatment:** Penile extenders.
Description: Device with proximal and distal fixation points designed to progressively stretch the penis. They can be worn under the clothing.
Potential benefits: There have been multiple studies published in peer reviewed literature suggesting gains of 1.3 to 1.8 cm.
Risks: Potential problems with skin irritation, erosion, and ulcers. Continuation of penile extenders.
Cost: $50-500

9:     **Treatment:** All-day stretch device
Description: A harness is placed over or under the glans and secured under tension to the leg or around the chest or waist. Constant steady tension is applied for extended periods of time.
Potential benefits: Application of traction promotes an increase in length.
Risks: Skin irritation, skin ulcer, temporary numbness.
Cost: $100-300

10:   **Treatment:** Penile weights
Description: A harness is attached to the shaft of the penis and weights are affixed to a hook apparatus on the harness.
Potential benefits: Aggressive form of traction therapy may increase length. Recommended by some surgeons after division of ligament.
Risks: Skin trauma, skin ulcer, bruising, discoloration, decreased sensation, erectile dysfunction.
Cost: $100-300

11:   **Treatment:** Injectable Collagen Zyderm, Zyplast.
Description: Bovine-linked collagen,; injected under the skin.
Potential benefit: Temporary, can be treated with Collagenase if there are side effects.
Risks: Small risk of allergic reaction, requires skin test prior to administration
Cost: $2,000

12: Treatment: Synthetic injectable collagen, Cosmoderm, Cosmoplast.
Description: Injectable product administered under the skin
Potential benefit: Temporary increase in girth of the shaft.
Risks: Temporary gains; may produce an irregular contour.
Cost: $2,500

13: Treatment: Hyaluronic acid fillers, Restylane, Perlane, Juvaderm.
Description: Injectable filler, widely used in cosmetic treatments.
Potential benefits: Stimulates collagen growth, can be reversed with hyaluronidase.
Risks: Only used for girth; will be temporary, typically less than 18 months.
Cost: $2,500-5,000

14: Treatment: PLLA Sculptra,NewFill.
Description: Injectable biodegradeable scaffold for collagen production.
Potential benefits: Increase in girth; replaced by patient's own natural collagen.
Risks: Potential bumps or granulomas develop years after treatment.
Cost: $3,000-50,000

15: Treatment: Calcium hydroxyapatite Radiesse or ArteFill.
Description: Injectable product absorbed by the body and replaced with natural collagen.
Potential benefits: Increase in girth; longer lasting than hyaluronic acid fillers.
Risks: Migration; temporary results.
Cost: $2,000-3,000

16: Treatment: Micronized alloderm, Megafill.
Description: Injectable biodegradeable scaffold
Potential benefit: Enhances girth; replaced by patient's natural tissues.
Risks: May migrate over the first six months.
Cost: $3,000-6,000

17: Treatment: Division of suspensory ligament, ligamentolysis.
Description: Surgical procedure under anesthesia; incision of ligament with scissors or laser.

Potential benefit: Increases length 1.5 to 2.5 c.m.; multiple series in peer reviewed literature.
Risks: Potential change in angle of erection, paradoxical subsequent retraction of the penis.
Cost: $3,000-$5,000

18: **Treatment:** Inverted VYplasty
Description: Employed during ligamentolysis to produce vertical lengthening of the skin.
Potential benefits: Facilitates lengthening of the penis.
Risks: Can create a dense scar or penile hump.
Cost: Included in price of ligamentolysis.

19: **Treatment:** Free fat transfer, FFT.
Description: Removal of fat either from around the penis (lower abdomen) or inner thighs, with transfer under the skin of the penis.
Potential benefit: May create allusion of longer penis by removal of fat around the penis; transfer of fat increases girth.
Risks: Irregular absorption of fat can create irregular, misshapen penis.
Cost: $4,000-10,000

20: **Treatment:** Dermal fat graft.
Description: A graft is usually taken from the crease under the buttocks. The epithelium is removed, and the graft is implanted above Buck's fascia , under the skin.
Potential benefits: Possible to create significant increase in girth.
Risks: Uncertain survival of the graft, which may contract. Additional risks of healing of the wound under the buttocks.
Cost: $4,000-10,000

21: **Treatment:** Allografts, Belladerm, Alloderm.
Description: Acellular scaffold derived from human skin replaced by natural tissues.
Potential benefits: Similar to dermal fat grafts; provides for girth without requiring an additional incision.
Risks: Delayed contraction; injury to overlying skin; necrosis; graft failure and infection.
Cost: $6,500-8,500

22:   Treatment: Elist implant.
Description: Soft silicone implant placed between Buck's fascia and the dartos fascia to increase girth.
Potential benefit: Permanent increase in girth.
Risks: Erosion; infection; wound problems; device may be palpable in some patients.
Cost: $12,000

23:   Treatment: Ventral phalloplasty.
Description: Surgical excision of scrotal web (tissue binding ventral surface of phallus to the scrotum).
Potential benefits: Presents the allusion of a longer penis; can be combined with insertion of a penile prosthesis.
Risks: Small risk of wound problem; does not increase stretched penile length.
Cost: $1,500

24:   Treatment: PRP platelet rich plasma.
Description: Platelet rich plasma, derived from the patient's own blood contains multiple growth factors which may help to regenerate penile tissue.
Potential benefits: May improve erectile function; may offer potential benefit when combined with mesenchymal stem cells in terms of growth.
Risks: Unproven benefit in reference to penile growth; no peer reviewed literature demonstrating gains in size.
Cost: $1,000-2,000

25:   Treatment: Clamping.
Description: Placing a clamp at the base of the penis during erection, preventing the venous outflow of blood.
Potential benefit: Increased length and girth.
Potential risks: If oxygen-depleted blood is trapped too long, potential injury to the corpora; risk of stricture formation in the urethra; lack of studies in peer reviewed literature.
Cost: $100-150

26:    **Treatment:** PLGA scaffold.

Description: Biodegradeable scaffold is placed surgically and cultured cells derived from the patient are used to populate the scaffold.

Potential benefits: The patient's own cells are utilized to create girth. Tissue engineering is the likely future of penile enlargement.

Risks: At this time, there is uncertain survival of the cultured cells, and the scaffold is somewhat rigid. Gains have not been permanent

Cost: $10,000-150,000

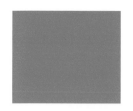

Glossary Of Terms

Alloderm: A regenerative tissue matrix, derived from the skin of cadavers used to augment girth,

Allograft: Tissue that is transplanted,from one person to another person (same species).

Anorgasmia: Persistent inability to achieve orgasm in spite of adequate sexual stimulation.

Belladerm: A regenerative tissue matrix, derived from surgical specimens of living donors.

BDD: Body dysmorphic disorder: A mental illness which results in obsession on a perceived flaw in appearance.

Cell Division: Division of a cell into two daughter cells. After division each daughter cell has the same genetic material and half of the cytoplasm.

cGMP: Cyclic Guanosine Monophosphate, acts as a second messenger, and in particular promotes increased blood flow to facilitate erections. Erection pills such as Viagra act by inhibiting the breakdown of cGMP by inhibiting PDE5.

Clitoris: The most sensitive erogenous zone in women, located cranial, or above the urethra. The glans of the clitoris is analogous to the glans of the penis, and contains more than 8,000 nerve endings.

Collagen: The main structural protein found in man. A tough, fibrous protein found in bone and soft tissue.

Contralateral: The opposite side relative to a structure or condition.

Corpora Cavernosa: Contain most of the blood in the penis during an erection; paired bodies that contain erectile tissue.

Corporal Disproportion: When the 2 corpora are of different sizes from one another the penis may bend of one side. When the corpora are of the same size, but disproportionate to the urethra, the penis may bend downwards.

Corpus Spongiosum: The spongy tissue that surrounds the urethra, and expands to form most of the glans penis distally.

Cytoplasm: The material within the cell. Increasing the cytoplasm is an essential part of growth.

Dartos Muscle: Also referred to as superficial fascia of the penis, lies just beneath the skin of the penis and above Buck's fascia.

Distal: Further from the center of the body, or point of attachment.

Dorsal: The back surface, in regards to the penis, as one looks down at the penis, it is the top side.

Dupytren's Contracture: A condition of the hand, a soft tissue disorder with tightening and thickening analogous to a condition of the penis known as Peyronie's disease.

Firbroblasts: A type of cell that produces matrix and collagen. The most common cell of connective tissue in humans.

Flaccid: Relaxed, loose, soft, the penis in the unexcited state.

Girth: The measurement around the penis, the circumference.

Glans: Also known as glans penis, or helmet. The bulbous structure at the end of the penis.

Glycosaminoglycans: GAG, polysaccharides that contain amino groups, occur as components of connective tissue.

Granuloma: A mass, or growth which can be caused by inflammation, infection, or any foreign body. A response of the immune system. A granuloma is a microscopic diagnosis demonstrating cells known as macrophages (or histiocytes).

Grower: Those who have a flaccid penis that grows significantly when stimulated.

G -spot: A sensitive area on the anterior wall of the lower one third of the vagina, first identified by Dr. Grafenberg. An erogenous area which may respond to sexual stimulation.

Hyaluronic Acid: HA is a glycosaminoglycan widely distributed throughout the body. A major component of skin and involved in repair of tissues. Among the most common fillers used in cosmetic facial injections.

Hypospadias: A congenital condition in which the urethral meatus is on the underside of the penis, rather than at the tip.

Jelq: A manual exercise in which an individual milks the blood in the penis forward with the intended purpose of promoting growth.

Kegel Exercise: An exercise designed to strengthen the pelvic floor musculature. The levator muscles are squeezed, resulting in contraction of the external urinary sphincter. This exercise is utilized by women to regain urinary control after childbirth. In men, this maneuver may force additional blood into the penis.

Lateral: From the side, or toward the side.

Lidocaine: A common short-acting local anesthetic agent. Also known as Xylocaine.

Ligamentolysis: Also known as division of the suspensory ligament. The most common surgical procedure utilized to promote increased penile length.

Lipoaspirate: The material removed at the time of liposuction. This material can subsequently be processed and used to increase penile girth.

Marcaine: A local anesthetic, longer last affect than Lidocaine. Also known as Bupivicaine.

Micropenis: A penis that is 2.75 inches or less in length, a condition found in .6% of men.

Narcissist: A personality disorder, in which the individual has an inflated sense of self- importance, self- involved, vain and selfish.

Necrosis: Death of cell tissue which is permanent.

Nitric Oxide (NO): A vasodilator that helps to mediate erections. Helps to activate increased cGMP levels, which in turn is a messenger for increased vascular flow to the penis.

Nodule: A swelling or collection of cells in the body, a lump or protuberance in the skin that can be felt.

Paraphimosis: A condition found in uncircumsised men, the foreskin is stuck proximal to the glans penis, and can't be pulled over the glans.

PDE5 Inhibitors: Include erection pills such as Viagra, Cialis, Levitra and Staxyn.

Petechia: A red or purple spot caused by bleeding into the skin

Peyronie's Disease: An acquired condition that results in the formation of plaques on the corpora cavernosa. This leads to shortening of the penis, bending of the penis, and pain with erections.

Phimosis: A condition found in uncircumcised men, the foreskin is stuck over the glans penis, and can't be retracted.

Proximal: Nearer to the center of the body. or point of attachment.

Regenerative Medicine: Includes tissue engineering and also self healing. Tissue engineering and regenerative medicine are very similar and are often used as interchangeable terms.

Scrotal Web: A web of tissue tethering the ventral surface of the penis to the scrotum, detracting from the perceived length of the penis.

Shower: A male with a large, flaccid penis that has limited growth.

SPL: Stretched penis length. Obtained by pressing a rule against the pubic bone, and measuring to the end of the penis.

SPS: Small penis syndrome. A condition in which one has a normal-sized penis but has disproportionate anxiety that their penis is too small.

Suspensory Ligament: The ligament which connects the penis to the pubis, Helps to maintain the angle of the penis during erections.

Taint: Also known as the perineum, the area bounded by the scrotum and anus, it ain't the scrotum, it ain't the anus.

Testosterone: Steroid hormone produced mainly by the testicles, but also by the adrenals. Stimulates penis growth prior to puberty. Responsible for secondary sexual charcteristics, and has a role in sexual desire and intercourse.

Tissue Engineering: The goal of which is to create functional forms that restore, maintain or improve damaged tissues or whole organs. Combines scaffolds, cells and biologically active molecules into living tissues.

Tunica Albuginea: The thick covering of the corpora cavernosa, helps to contain the erectile tissue.

Urethra: The tubular structure responsible for transport of urine and ejaculate.

Urethral Meatus: The distal opening of the urethra, the pee hole.

Ventral: The underside, in reference to the penis, the side that faces the body when the penis is flaccid.

Verapamil: A calcium channel blocker, sometimes injected into Peyronie's plaques to help dissolve them.

Vitiligo: A skin condition in which there is a loss of skin color in blotches, due to loss of skin pigment cells.

Xenograft: Tissue transplanted from one species to another species (a pig valve)

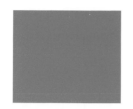

References

Chapter 1. References.

1. Simoniski, K and Bain, J (1993) The relationship among height, penile length, and foot size. Ann. Sex Res 6:231-235

2. Guthrie, Smith,Graham. Testosterone treatment for micropenis during early childhood, The Journal Of Pediatrics, August 1973.

3. M Francine A.B., Van de Wiel, H.B.M,, Weijmer Schultz W.CM . What importance to women attribute to the size of the penis, European urology, November 2002 Vol. 42(5).

4. Grafenberg,Ernest The role of the urethra in female orgasm. The International Journal of Sexology, February 1950

5. Eisenman,Russell Penis size: Survey of female perceptions of sexual satisfaction,BMC Women's Health 2001, 1:1

6. Lever,Janet; Frederick,David;Peplau,Letitia Anne Psychology of Men & Masculinity,Vol 7(3), Jul 2006, 129-143

7. Blanchard,R and Bogaert,A.F (1996) File demographic comparisons of homosexual and heterosexual man in the Kinsey interview data. Arch. Sex Behavior 25:551-579

8. Grov, Christian, Parsons Jeffery T. The association between penis size in sexual health among men who have sex with men, Archives of sexual behavior, June 2010 volume 39 issue 3, 788-797

Chapter 2 references.

1. Jamison,Gebhard. Penis size increase between flaccid and erect states, analysis of the Kinsey data. The journal of sex research. Volume 24 issue 1 1988

2. Kinsey,Pomeroy,Martin Sexual behavior in the human male,1948

3. Francken, Van de Weil,Can Driel. What importance do women a tribute to the size of the penis. European urology 2002 volume 42

4. Andreason Bardach. Dysmorphobia: symptom or disease? The American Journal of psychiatry volume 134(6) June 1977

5. Cask,Keating,Miranda-Sousa,Carrion. Ventral Phalloplasty, Asian journal of andrology,January 2008l

Chapter 3 references

1. Schwarzenegger, Klotz,Reifenrath, The prevalence of Peyronie's disease; results of a large survey. British Journal of urology international 2001. Vol 88. 727-730

2. Brooks, James D. Anatomy of the lower urinary tract and male genitalia, Campbell-Walsh Urology, ninth edition,

3. Lue, Tom F, Physiology of penile erection and pathophysiology of erectile dysfunction, Campbell-Walsh Urology, ninth edition

4. Savior, Kim, Soliway A prospective study measuring penile length in men treated with radical prostatectomy for prostate cancer. The journal of urology April 2003 vol 169(4)

5. Mundind, Wessells,Dalkin. Pilot study of changes in stretched penile length three months after radical retropubic prostatectomy. Urology October 2001volume 58(4)

6. Koehler,Pedro,Hendlin,Utz,Ugarte. A pilot study on the early use of the vacuum erection device after radical retropubic prostatectomy British Journal of urology international. 2007

7. Frank, Anderson,Rubinstein. Frequency of sexual dysfunction in normal couples. The New England Journal of medicine. July 20, 1978

8. Laumann, Paik, Rosen. Sexual dysfunction in the United States prevalence and predictors. Journal of the American medical Association February 10, 1999

Chapter 4 references

1. Davis,Michael. Herbal remedies: adverse effects and drug interactions. International essential tremor foundation

2. Palmer,Ashton,Moncada Vascular endothelial cells synthesize nitric oxide from L-arginine. Nature. 333 664-666

3. Grundy,Lena Vega, McGovern Efficacy safety and tolerability of once daily niacin for the treatment of dyslipidemia associated with type two diabetes. Journal of the American medical Association July 22, 2002

4. Schaumburg,Kaplan,Windebank. Sensory neuropathy from pyridoxine abuse,The New England Journal of Medicine August 25, 1983

5. Chandra, excessive intake of zinc in pairs immune responses, Journal of the American medical Association September 21 ,1984

6. Morales,Condra, Owen Is Yohimbine effective in the treatment of organic impotency? Results of a controlled trial. The journal of urology 1987, 137(6)

7. Rohdewald. A review of the French maritime pine bark extract (Pycnogenol) a herbal medication with a diverse clinical pharmacology. International Journal of clinical pharmacology and therapeutics 2002 40(4).

8. Cyrus, Nicolis,Moinard. Almost all about citrulline in mammals. Amino acids. August 2005

9. Wiseman, Propionyl-L-Carnitine Drugs and aging, March 1998 volume 12 issue 3

10. Karin, Tongkat Ali A review on its ethnobotany and pharmacological importance. Phytotherapy, October 2010 volume 81 (7)

11. Wilt, Ishani, Stark. Saw palmetto extract for treatment of benign prostatic hyperplasia a systemic review. Journal of the American medical association,November 11, 1998

12. Gauthaman, Adaiken. Aphrodisiac properties of. Tribulus Terrestris. extract in normal and castrated rats. Life sciences August 9, 2002

13. Richards,Smitasiri,Jeenapongsa. Butea superba enhances penile erection in rats. Phytotherapy research. April 18, 2006

14. Delivery, Burke, Palmer. The affects of deer antler velvet extract on aerobic power, erythropoiesis and muscular strength and endurance characteristics. The Journal of sports nutrition and exercise metabolism 2003. 251-265.

15. Heck,DeWitt,Luke's. Potential interactions between alternative therapies and warfarin. American Journal of health system pharmacy July 1, 2000

16. Dunks,Walczak. Collagen hydrolysate as a new diet supplement Scientific bulletin of the technical University of Lodz. No 1058. Bol 73

Chapter 6 references

1. Bosshardy,Farwek,Sikora. Objective measurement of the effectiveness, therapeutic success and dynamic mechanisms of the vacuum device. British Journal urology international. Vol 75, issue 6

2. Collin,Artini,Scroppo,Mancini,Castiglioni. International journal of impotence research. volume 14 supplement

3. Nowroost, Amini,Ayati,Jamshidian,Radkhah. Applying extender devices in patients with penile dysmorphophobia; assessment of tolerability, efficacy and impact on erectile function.   Journal of sexual medicine, 2015

Chapter 7 references

1. Prockop,Kivirikko,Tuderman The biosynthesis of collagen and it's disorders. The New England Journal of Medicine July 5, 1979
2. Hanke, Higley,Jolivette. Abscess formation and local necrosis after treatment with Zyderm or Zyplast collagen implant. Journal of the American Academy of Dermatology August 1991
3. Bentkover The biology of facial fillers. Facial plastic surgery volume 25 number 2. 2009
4. Friedman, Mafong,Kauvar. Safety data of injectable non-animal stabilized hyaluronic acid gel for soft tissue augmentation augmentation
5. Maloney,Murphy, Cole. Cymetra. Facial plastic surgery 2004 volume 20(2)
6. Scalds I. What we have learned about soft tissue augmentation over the past 10 years. Journal of the American medical association facial plastic surgery classics
7. Kim,Kwak, Jeon. Human glans penis augmentation using injectable hyaluronic acid gel. International Journal of impotence research The journal of sexual medicine June 12, 2002

Chapter 8 references

1. Li, Kaye,Kell. Penile suspensory ligament division for penile augmentation : indications and results European urology April 2006 volume 49(4)
2. Wylie,Eardley. Penile size in the small penis syndrome. British Journal of urology international March 12, 2007
3. Khomeini, Eisenmann-Klein, Cardoso, CooleyKacher,Gombos,Baker Brava Autologous fat transfer is a safe and effective breast augmentation alternative
4. Schiffman,Mirrafati. Fat transfer techniques; The effect of harvest and transfer methods on adipocyte liability,a review of the literature 7 July 2008
5. Bruno, Senderoff, Fracchis. Reconstruction of penile wounds following complications of AlloDerm based augmentation phalloplasty. Plastic and reconstructive surgery January 2007 volume 119(1)

6. Martin,Parker. Penile length alterations following penile prosthesis surgery. European urology April 2007 volume51(4).

7. Austoni,Guarneri, Cassaniga. A new technique for augmentation phalloplasty ; albugineal surgery with bilateral saphenous grafts-three years of experience. European urology September 2002

8. Kaufman, Miller,Huang. Fat transfer for facial recontouring; is there science behind the art? Plastics and reconstructive surgery. June 2007 volume 119 issue 7